MAN UP!

MAN UP!

Paul O'Donnell

ARTISAN
NEW YORK

Published by Artisan
A division of Workman Publishing Company, Inc.
225 Varick Street
New York, NY 10014-4381
artisanbooks.com

Published simultaneously in Canada by Thomas Allen & Son, Limited

Library of Congress Cataloging-in-Publication Data
O'Donnell, Paul, 1961–
Man up! / Paul O'Donnell.
p. cm.
Includes index.
ISBN 978-1-57965-391-0
1. Men—Life skills guides. I. Title.
HQ1090.O334 2011
646.70081—dc22   2010039447

Design by Robert Perino

Printed in China

7 9 10 8

Contents

Introduction

Man up. It's a challenge to a guy to be his best. Be a man. What does it mean? A man, a guy, a dude is a male of whatever age, shape, or occupation, understood by what he has in common with all other males. That includes a lot of the stereotypes from our grandfathers' days: A man is decisive, gallant, capable, competitive, rational. He's adaptable: sometimes he runs with the pack, other times he strikes out on his own; he's a partner in some situations and a leader in others. He's a philosopher and a mechanic. He's a son, a boyfriend, a wingman, the brains *and* the muscle, self-sufficient *and* a man of the world. More than ever, guys are expected to know how to dress themselves, how to throw a raucous party, how to feather their nest for nights at home—alone or with company.

Who expects all this of modern guys? These days, guys are expecting it of themselves.

What makes all this business of being a guy possible is confidence. With the conviction that confidence is better learned than assumed, I've written this book with the help of many tutors. Some are men in my own life: friends, brothers, fathers of friends, bartenders. I've talked to state troopers and stunt drivers, brewers, poets, waiters, fashion editors, and salesmen. Not everyone I've interviewed is credited—many preferred not to be; some didn't know their expertise was being sought for the purpose of this book. In any event, there is hardly an entry that comes from the advice of just one person.

The tips are broken into chapters according to the situations, expected and unexpected, that guys find themselves in: at work, in a bar, at home in bed, or climbing mountains. I don't presume to teach everything anyone needs to know about sailing a boat or ordering wine or swimming. Instead I've tried to give readers a basic concept to build on, or detailed one skill that, I hope, will transform an everyday activity into an enriching experience. I've paid special attention to dealing with difficult situations—from flat tires to a night in jail. There are few hard-and-fast rules in life, but nothing is as difficult as it seems if you know a couple of basic techniques or principles. I don't guarantee that this book will pull you through every chapter of your life without a scratch, but I hope it will give you the confidence to handle what's coming next.

MAN UP!

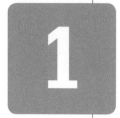

1

Brand: Me

Get a look at your reflection. Not just in the mirror:
Take a listen to your phone greeting. Review the last
five texts you sent. Check out the clothes hanging in
your closet.

How you present yourself has a powerful influence
on where and how far you go in life. It's not just how
you dress either or what picture you stick on
your online profile. You reveal yourself through

your table manners, your friendships and how you conduct them, the music leaking from your headphones. Think of every encounter as another expression of the person you want to project, and ultimately want to be: your personal brand.

FIRST IMPRESSIONS

1 Which hairstyle is right for me?

A guy's coif should not look like he spends forever lingering over it. Neat or messy, shaggy-locked rock star or buzz-cut Semper Fi, your hair should balance practicality and sheer indifference.

Remember looks can be deceiving. Extremely short hair requires frequent barber visits; long hair keeps you out of the barber chair, but means constant shampooing and brushing. And don't let a Goth's mess of jet black locks fool you: the dude spends more time swapping hair-dyeing tips than your grandmother. When picking a style, think about how much time you want to budget for hair care, from a little a day to an hour or so once a week. And using the list below as a guide, consider how your hairstyle works with the shape of your head and face.

▶ **BALD** Confident and virile, bald heads favor smooth, round craniums and square faces. Bald is the manly way out if you're losing your hair, and is much, much better than trying to rock a comb-over. (See page 7.)

▶ **BUSINESSMAN'S CUT** Conservative but with a little length at the sides, this one's good for faces wider at the jaw. It's

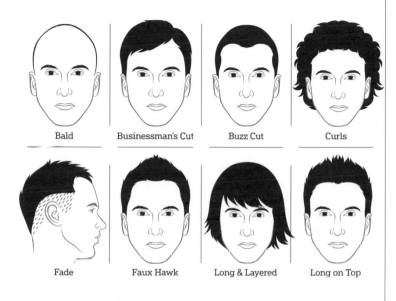

Bald	Businessman's Cut	Buzz Cut	Curls
Fade	Faux Hawk	Long & Layered	Long on Top

perfect for the guy who needs to look professional and clean-cut every day, without having to spend too much effort beyond combing it into place. Let your sideburns reach the bottom of your ears, and you'll be sporting a **Jeff Gordon.**

▶ **BUZZ CUT** The shorter you keep your buzz these days, the edgier you look, but you'll never look less than neat.

▶ **CURLS** Let them bush out to lend height to a square face or a short frame. Curls can be well groomed—picture Seth Rogen on the red carpet—or out of control—see Seth Rogen in any of his movies.

DIY

2 How do I get punk colors?

You can install a raging blue, pink, or purple punk hairdo at a tony salon and still retain your street cred. But you can also get Day-Glo to go using professional materials and methods at home. It's always good to have another pair of hands, so ask a pal for an assist, and follow these steps:

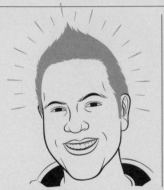

1

BLEACH
Get a professional white bleach-and-developer mix at a beauty supply store—a number-10 strength for blonds; number 40 for dark hair—and gunk it on. If a regular drugstore is all you have access to, look for a kit with words like "super extra blonding."

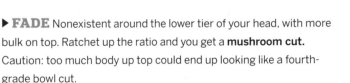

▶ **FADE** Nonexistent around the lower tier of your head, with more bulk on top. Ratchet up the ratio and you get a **mushroom cut.** Caution: too much body up top could end up looking like a fourth-grade bowl cut.

▶ **FAUX HAWK** Clipped merely short on the sides with a long, shaggy stripe down the middle, this modified Mohawk keeps your locks tamed for work and easy to spike for a wilder look.

4

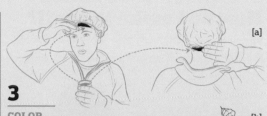

2

BLOW-DRY
Snap on a shower cap and dry your hair through it, *keeping the dryer moving* in small circles. The darker the color you want, the longer you dry.

3

COLOR
Rub Vaseline around your hairline and on your ears to keep the dye from coloring your skin. Using a specifically designed hair-color brush you also bought at the beauty store, paint the dye on your bleached locks for at least ten minutes, getting as little on your scalp as possible.

4

RINSE
Wash the dye from your hair per the instructions on the box, and enjoy your new alterna-look while it lasts.

▶ **LONG AND LAYERED** This style can go shaggy and blended for a Justin Bieber look or chunky for an all-American feel. A saltwater-washed version that's all bangs is called **surfer hair.**

▶ **LONG ON TOP** Tidy around the back and ears but something to play with on top, this style adds length to a round face, or—throw in a little hair gunk and tousle it at the front—softens a receding hairline. For extra style, comb it back in a gelled wave for a **pompadour.**

1
2
3
4
5
6

3 Tapered or squared: How do I make the call?

Haircutters will often ask how you want your hair at the neckline in the back, tapered or squared off. Tapered is the neater and longer lasting option, but guys with a skinny neck might want the hairline to be squared off (sometimes called blocked) to add the illusion of width. A tapered back, on the other hand, slims a thick neck.

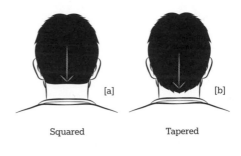

[a] Squared
[b] Tapered

4 Do I really need to use conditioner?

Yes. Shampoo can't distinguish between good oil and bad oil, so it strips it all out, leaving your hair dry, limp, and damaged. Conditioner restores the luster. Can't spare the time to let it sink in? The bulk of the goo's work is done in the first minute. Shampoo and rinse, massage the conditioner into your hair, and keep your head out of the water's way while you soap up the rest of you. By the time you're finished, you can rinse it out. If your hair is naturally oily, condition once or twice a week instead of every day.

Ten truths about going bald

1 No woman will leave you or refuse to sleep with you because you're balding.

2 More hair doesn't make you look younger.

3 You may get results from Rogaine, but eventually your girlfriend will find the box.

4 Hairpieces and comb-overs make an enemy of many beautiful things in life, like a midnight swim, a summer breeze, and fingers through your hair.

5 Clean-shaven heads are no longer restricted to Batman's archenemies and circus strongmen.

6 Your hair loss is the result of an excess of testosterone, literally the essence of manliness.

7 Balding men look smarter.

8 The balder you are, the less prone you are to a bad hair day or hat-head.

9 Forty percent of men show signs of balding by age 35, and 65 percent by age 65.

10 There are no bald politicians.

5 Should I let my hair go gray?

Some guys start to go gray before they are thirty; for some it never happens. If you start to spot gray hairs and it bothers you, there are some things you can do. First, ask a professional hairstylist for advice. Any pro worth his or her salt will respond by listing the stars (Patrick Dempsey) and serious players (Anderson Cooper) who have allowed themselves to go gray. If you still want it gone, let a stylist give you a credible dye job for as natural a look as possible.

1
2
3
4
5
6

6 **How do I shave?**

Many guys learned their method from their fathers, who learned from their dads, as a sort of tribal rite. As a result, most shaving routines involve a fair amount of witchcraft. The science of shaving requires just two essential elements: heat and moisture.

Start by dousing your face four or five times with water that's as hot as you can stand. Add soap, scrub up, and rinse. After this treatment, your whiskers should be as soft as a kitten's fur and bristling for the blade. Maintain their upright attitude by applying shaving cream from bottom to top, against the grain of your beard. You don't need a lot of cream: just enough to keep the water on your skin and to lubricate the blade.

Shave the wide-open spaces of your cheeks first, to give the water and shaving cream more time to soak into the tougher hair around your mouth and chin. Keep your skin taut by stretching it gently with the fingers of your free hand (some guys achieve this by filling their cheeks with air). Use short, smooth strokes and dip the blade frequently in hot water.

Proceed no farther than your clavicle, also known as your collarbone. Everything else is chest hair. There is no upper limit to your shaving area—if it looks like a whisker, shave it. If you have hair growing between your eyebrows, define them with a quick shave.

Purists insist you should only shave downward, arguing that shaving in any direction except the one your whiskers grow in causes ingrown hairs. It's a rare guy, however, whose every last whisker grows in any one direction; most faces feature swirls, flanking maneuvers, and divots (for instance, the philtrum, that indent on your upper lip). So if you need to shave from several angles, by all means do so.

You're finished when your skin feels smooth when you run your fingers across it. Rinse your face and dry it with a towel, making sure you've left no shaving cream under your ears.

Finally, apply moisturizer to prevent irritation and razor burn.

7 **What type of razor is for me?**

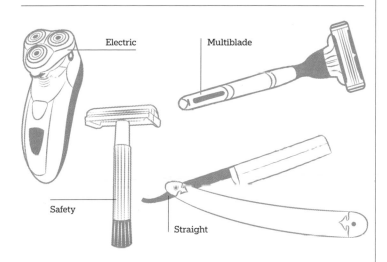

Electric

Multiblade

Safety

Straight

▶ **ELECTRIC** With a gently humming gadget that slides painlessly across your skin, without the mess of soap and water, it's almost like you aren't shaving at all. Unfortunately, you're almost not: electrics reduce your beard to a stubble, but don't approach the closeness of a regular razor. Electrics are better for maintaining the fashionably gruff look of a few days' growth, and are just the thing for trimming a beard or mustache.

▶ **MULTIBLADE** Perhaps only the Pentagon spends more on R&D than the highly competitive major razor companies, whose flexible designs are aimed at turning the complex topography of your face into an easily maneuvered flat surface. Their advertising campaigns tout comfort, but their true advantage is speed.

Experts say that any more than three blades don't measurably improve closeness or comfort, and they generally pooh-pooh "comfort strips" and other gizmos. Let your fancy be your guide, but keep a multiblade, swiveling razor in your arsenal.

▶ **SAFETY RAZOR** Your grandfather used one of these contraptions built to hold double-edged blades before the invention of cartridge razors. Nowadays some guys are reviving them, not only for their retro chic, but, at about $40 for a basic model—try a German maker for their precision engineering—with blades around 60 cents apiece, to save not a small amount of money over time. Getting a close, nick-free shave takes more time and a little practice, but fans say the safety razor turns shaving into a contemplative, self-pampering treat.

▶ **STRAIGHT RAZOR** Every guy should get a professional shave with a straight razor once in his life—less for the shave itself, than to experience the ideal of what a shave can be: a pampering, hot-towel-laden spa. An old-school barber may oblige you if you ask, but a safer bet is to visit one of the men's "lounges" that have been enjoying a vogue recently, which specialize in throwback deluxe services.

8 WHAT DO I PUT ON MY FACE TO SHAVE?

PIROOZ SARSHAR
cofounder of the Grooming Lounge, Washington, D.C.

"I don't recommend a shaving cream that comes out of the can that turns into a big foam on your face. Most of the foam doesn't touch your skin, rendering it useless, and a foam doesn't provide enough lubrication to give you a comfortable shave. The best type of shave cream goes on clear, so you can see the hair you're trying to shave off, and that creates a smooth surface for the razor to glide on. If you're trawling the aisles in a drugstore, look for a shaving cream that is rich in glycerin. But if you want the ultimate shave, use a natural shaving oil, which uses the same oils you find in your kitchen, like sesame oil or olive oil, but has been developed to suspend your beard and clean up more easily. You can find them online and in some big-box stores."

9 Do I need to use a shaving brush?

Shaving brushes look antiquated but have yet to be bettered as a method of applying shaving cream. The bristles exfoliate dead skin cells as they coat your beard and make the whiskers stand up. Use badger hair, which is durable enough for extended use, but soft enough for your face to stand daily.

10 How do I stop a shaving cut?

Rinse the cut with clean cold water as you would any small cut. If you are old school, you'll have a styptic pencil on hand. Wet the tip and smudge it gently against the cut. A moist alum block, rubbed on the cut or across your whole shaving area, will also soothe everything in its path.

If you don't have one of these handy, tear off a fragment of facial tissue or toilet paper, just enough to cover the cut, and stick it to the cut while it's relatively blood-free. Keep the tissue there until it is completely dry. Remove with care so as not to reopen the cut.

11 What can I use when I forget my shaving cream?

Use hair conditioner. It won't lather, but it will keep your beard soft and your skin slick while you get a decent shave.

12 How do I pick a moisturizer?

Even if you don't have especially dry skin, it's important to moisturize to keep your skin healthy, and to apply sunblock every day.

Pick a moisturizer made for your skin type. If your skin is dry and sensitive, use a super-hydrating moisturizer with glycerin and vitamin E, and steer clear of fragrances, which can irritate sensitive skin. If your skin is oily and acne-prone, you need an oil-free moisturizer, or even one that contains clay or salicylic acid to soak up excess oil. Some guys are oily in places and dry in others; there's nothing wrong with applying two types of moisturizer in the right places. Use a moisturizer that comes with sunscreen of at least SPF 15.

13 **What kind of facial hair should I grow?**

Whiskers do more than give you an excuse not to shave. They influence the contours of your face—not to mention the attitude you emit.

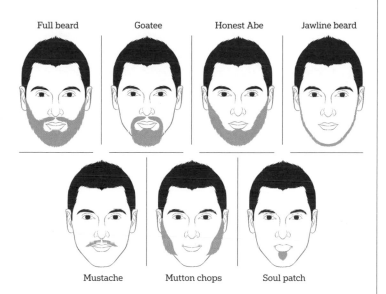

| Full beard | Goatee | Honest Abe | Jawline beard |

| Mustache | Mutton chops | Soul patch |

▶ **FULL BEARD** Fine for men of any profession except cops and bank officers, beards hide a weak chin, conceal heavy jowls, and convey friendliness, frankness, and a woolly thoughtfulness. The full beard is also the lowest maintenance facial do, but requires the most patience to grow. Allow four weeks for plush coverage; the longer you keep it, the better a beard looks—with regular trimming, of course.

▶ **GOATEE** This mustache/Vandyke beard combo lengthens a wide face and awards an already long face a look of brooding passion. Once considered professorial, goatees became ubiquitous —and a bit trite—among hipsters in the 1990s. Its popularity continues, perhaps because even light-bearded guys can grow a passably robust goatee.

▶ **HONEST ABE OR OLD DUTCH** A beard with no mustache has been popular for years in rural areas, either with peaks climbing over the chin or neatly tucked under the jawline. A strong look lately for indie musicians.

▶ **JAWLINE BEARD** The thinner the line of whiskers, the more urban this style of beard looks. A jawliner accentuates your face's bone structure; so if yours is not great, don't go here.

▶ **MUSTACHE** Match the proportions of your 'stache to your face—broad ones for wide faces, finer ones for finer features—but contrast the ends: rounded ends for square faces and square ends for round faces. As a rule you should fill the space between nose and mouth. Go beyond it, and you're a renegade ("gringo," "Fu Manchu"); fall short and you're a lounge lizard (pencil-thin) or a porn star (tightly trimmed away from both lip and nose).

▶ **MUTTONCHOPS** Sideburns extending below the corners of the mouth convey a sort of hillbilly pride. Hitch them to your mustache and you're wearing "the Franz Josef," named after a fastidious early-twentieth-century Austrian duke.

▶ **SOUL PATCH** Jazz horn players sported spit catchers below their bottom lips to catch their drool as they blew. Today's chin spinach varies in location, but still reads as jazzman bohemian.

14 **How do I trim my mustache?**

Use a good pair of mustache scissors, which gives you more control over what you're cutting than an electric trimmer does. Wet your 'stache a little and, with a fine-toothed comb, brush the hairs down. Clip slowly and conservatively or you may end up having to shave it off entirely to, uh, save face.

15 **Should I get a manicure?**

Sure, but the question is where. Although full-service salons for men are a growing trend in urban areas, most guys have access only to woman-dominated nail joints. If you brave it, get a manicure with everything but polish (even clear lacquer looks garish on a male hand). Or next time you go on vacation, visit a spa and ask for a manicure as part of your pampering.

Meanwhile, perform due diligence at home. Wash your hands with plenty of soap and rinse. Grab your nailbrush—a short, soft-bristled one with two short handles that curl around your fingers—and rub the bristles into a bar of soap. With soapy bristles perpendicular to your fingers, scrub across your fingernail tops until they are shining. If the brush can't get every last bit of dirt, use your nail clipper to shorten the nail until the brush can reach it. To make sure your nails look neat (and short enough to clean them effectively), keep the white edge at the tip of the nail no more than a sixteenth of an inch long.

16 **Should I sculpt my body hair?**

"Manscaping," the practice of shaving, waxing, or creaming off a guy's body hair, has gone mainstream, perhaps because more guys (and their girlfriends) are watching more depilated porn stars lately, or because hairless pectorals and biceps (and genitals) look bigger. Women accustomed to scrubbing hair from various areas of their bodies may have come to expect their dudes to denude themselves, too.

If it's your home slice who wants you bare to the skin, you don't have much more to say than, "I will if you will." Turn it into a private party for two: take turns shaving each other, or spreading the depilatory cream. (Have plenty of soothing lotion on hand, and celebrate with a drink *afterwards*, not before you take razor to body parts.)

You don't have to wait for a partner, or be maximally ripped, to experiment with a hair-free physique. Any hair you take off will grow back in a few weeks, and short of looking a little funny when it first comes back in, you'll do yourself no harm by using a depilatory cream or a razor. The same techniques apply to shaving body hair as shaving your face: prep with hot water and soap; use a clear, non-drying gel instead of foam (especially important around sensitive areas whose folds and clefts you're not used to shaving) and follow your shave with a moisturizer.

If you find you feel much happier hair-free, you might want to consider laser hair removal. These treatments are expensive, so pick an area—a lot of guys start with their back—where you long to get rid of unwanted hair permanently.

DRESSING WELL

17 **Can I wear pink?**

Dick Cheney does, and so does Kanye. Why shouldn't you? A pink dress shirt under a blazer or a suit is a springtime alternative to white. A pink linen number worn with khaki pants on a summer day is also an attractive choice. Not that pink can't make a statement: a pink polo shirt is the universally recognized preppy flag; pink canvas pants with an untucked shirt make you an artistic soul, while pink socks with a suit signals that a freethinker lurks beneath your conservative mien.

EXPERT WITNESS

18 HOW DO I ADD MORE STYLE TO MY LOOK?

COLBY McWILLIAMS
former head of men's fashion for luxury retailer Neiman Marcus

"There's no way to teach style. You have to try new things—get them into the fitting room and see what you're comfortable wearing. Start simply—less is usually best. You can be beautifully dressed and simply dressed. Stick with dark colors and solid shirts.

"This is easier to do when you're going to work, not as obvious when you're going casual. Men often react to casual settings by wearing everything baggy and pleated. You can upgrade your style just by paying attention to the volume of what you're wearing. Look for shirts that are a little fitted—even when you're wearing them with the tails out. In jeans, go with a straight leg and slimmer cut. Then use a jacket—one with plenty of pockets to store your phone and the rest of the stuff we carry these days—to pull everything together, even in casual situations."

19 **When do I wear shirts that need cuff links?**

Shirts with French cuffs, as the cuff-link-ready style is known, are completely acceptable anytime you wear a jacket. The only faux pas is letting your cuffs, now weighted with metal, protrude flamboyantly from your jacket sleeves. When buying French cuffs, get the sleeve length right, so that only a half inch is exposed when your jacket is on.

> **Tip:** If you're not used to the way cuff links clasp, practice attaching the cuff links to your sleeves before you put on your shirt.

20 **How do I dress to look slimmer?**

It may seem counterintuitive, but you'll look slimmer in clothes that are close-fitting. Buy jackets that are bigger in the shoulders and trim at the waist and pants that define your shape, even where you've got a few extra pounds. Avoid anything that billows or balloons: pleats and deep breaks on your pants only expand your profile. Make sure your belt is large enough to contain your waistline at its widest point; if your belly hangs over your pants, it accentuates your girth.

21 **How do I wear a hat?**

When it comes to hats, modern history is divided into Before JFK and After JFK. During his 1960 campaign, the young presidential contender went about half dressed—at least for his era—with neither a hat nor an overcoat, reputedly to emphasize his youth and vigor. The sight of the bareheaded swinger-politician, at least according to fashion legend, killed the hat as a necessary accessory.

Ironically, the hat is now coming back as a symbol of youthful nonchalance. The shapes of today's hipster headgear hark back to 1950s Rat Pack style, but the hat owes its rebirth to the ordinary baseball cap. Everybody looks good in a hat—you only need to find the lid that fits you. Here are some choices:

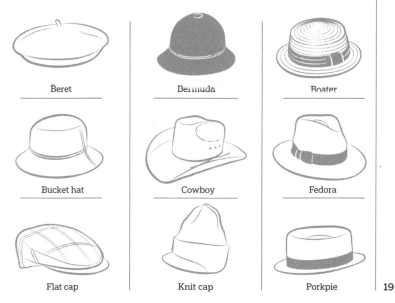

Beret	Bermuda	Boater
Bucket hat	Cowboy	Fedora
Flat cap	Knit cap	Porkpie

1
2
3
4
5
6

▶ **BERET** Don't worry about looking like a French poseur when you don one of these eminently practical toppers. The simple circle of wool adapts to any head, while its loft is a hedge against the dreaded hat-head. Just don't grow a shrimpy mustache and smoke butts backward, and you'll be fine.

▶ **BERMUDA** With old-school rap gaining cachet, the early rappers' topper, a pith helmet rendered in soft wool or cotton, is popping up again.

▶ **BOATER** A stiff straw hat with a flat brim and low, round crown, it has few legitimate uses outside productions of *Mary Poppins*— even on a boat.

▶ **BUCKET** In khaki or wool, the default rain hat for the commuter set.

▶ **COWBOY** Never out of style but strongly regional, the cattleman's cover should be worn casually in brown, white, or black, but only in white or cream with a suit. Urban guys should only wear one to bars with mechanical bulls.

▶ **FEDORA** Any film noir buff knows that the fedora, a brimmed hat whose crown is pinched on both sides in the front, was once as much a part of a man's look as his hair. Indiana Jones and the Blues Brothers rekindled the fedora's popularity, but mostly in casual contexts.

The broad-brimmed, felt version called a **trilby** is so deeply associated with 1940s movie detectives that wearing one with a suit makes cracks about Bogie (that's Humphrey Bogart) inevitable. In the summertime, however, a straw trilby with a casual shirt and khakis, or even shorts, is a cool play.

▶ **FLAT CAP** A conservative but quietly manly choice, this round cap with a stiff, barely visible brim blends with almost any look. Its more outlandish, flouncier cousin is the newsboy.

▶ **KNIT CAP** The traditional ski hat got an edgy twist when nineties grunge-rock groups adopted it, apparently as an alternative to showering. Lately the look has been updated by the addition of a brim to a loosely knitted version.

▶ **PORKPIE** This short-brimmed, flat-topped number has come to stand for a relaxed hipness. The version with a diamond-shaped crown is known as a four-corners.

22 **What are the rules for matching clothes?**

If you're color-challenged, or just don't have time to think of what goes with what, operate under these few simple rules:

▶ **MAKE SOLID CHOICES** Wear classic colors—navy and light blue, charcoal gray, tan, pink, red, and deep brown—and stick to solid shirts and suits.

1
2
3
4
5
6

Four looks for any occasion

Keeping the following four basic outfits in your closet is the sartorial equivalent of stocking a full bar.

1 | **NAVY SUIT** Combined with a white shirt, a dark red or maroon tie, and black cap-toe oxfords, this getup covers you for formal dinners, weddings, and professional power plays.

2 | **BLUE BLAZER AND GRAY PANTS** With a red-and-blue rep tie, this classic American look is a workday fallback; skip the tie, and you're set for your parents' house party. On friendlier turf, swap out the slacks for jeans. So versatile is this setup that many guys have a flannel blazer for cool months and a tropical-weight number for summer.

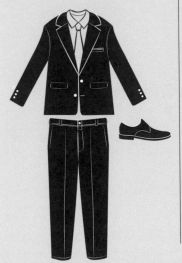

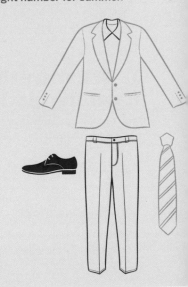

3 | CREWNECK SWEATER AND KHAKIS Once strictly a preppy ensemble, this look has been adopted by movie stars and indie rockers as the uniform for an off-day slouch. There are no rules for this combo: wear your collar and your shirttail in or out, or substitute faded jeans or cargoes. If you are tapped for an unexpected meet-up or impromptu dinner, tuck everything in and drag a comb through your hair.

4 | BLACK SHIRT AND DARK JEANS Every guy looks great with his face and hair set into relief by a black button-down shirt. The black palette lends a formal touch for parties or a first date, while the jeans keep the look relaxed. Give the outfit a solid base with lace-up ankle boots. Spin it fashion-forward with dark denim. In the summer, substitute a black polo shirt or black tee.

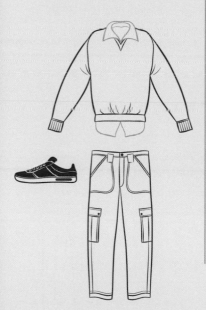

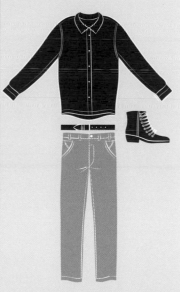

▶ **UNIFY YOUR LEATHERS** Your watchband, belt, and shoes should be of the same general color—brown with brown (or cordovan), black with black—and class: Don't mix a casual belt (cowboy, woven) with dress shoes.

▶ **CONTRAST COLORS** Matching your colors doesn't mean picking from the same palette. You don't want to be a symphony of beiges, or pair colors too close on the color chart (like black and navy, or orange and pink). Instead, oppose a dark suit with a white shirt, navy with pink, or brown with light blue.

▶ **TIE IN YOUR JACKET** A suit or sport jacket adds more elements to match, but no sweat: just make sure your tie has one color in common with your jacket, and your shirt and pants will work fine. With a tan jacket, for instance, wear a tie that contains tan, then contrast with a blue shirt.

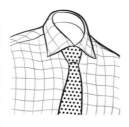

▶ **SHIRTS AND SKINS** Pay attention to what you wear directly next to your skin. If your complexion is dark, don't wear a brown shirt; if you're pale and blond, stay away from yellow. Instead, set off your complexion with a complementary color. Hint: blue complements nearly every skin tone, as does plain white.

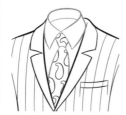

▶ **SIZE MATTERS** Color isn't the only thing to coordinate. You need to keep patterns in line as well, and your watchword here, too, is contrast. Match big with little. A small check on your shirt demands a large figure, like paisleys, on your tie; a large check plays well with a small dot.

23 **How do I de-stink my shoes?**

Bacteria lend shoes that distinctive aroma, and bacteria thrive on moisture. Most store-bought odor removers are desiccating agents—powders or charcoal grit that absorb the moisture in your shoes, but you can also remove the laces, splaying your shoes open, and set them in the sun. Dusting them lightly with baking soda will also dry them, as will a sachet of kitty litter. (Wrap the litter in a gauze bandage and tie it up with a rubber band.) Once the insides of the shoes are dry, dampen a cloth with rubbing alcohol and swab the interiors of your shoes to kill any remaining bacteria.

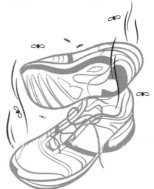

24 **Do I need an undershirt?**

Layers are key to staying warm, and also to staying cool. A cotton tee next to your skin absorbs sweat that would otherwise get mopped up by your shirt or sweater, which is not designed for the work. Undershirts help buffer your outer layer from all manner of odors and oils given off by your skin. An undershirt can also be an impromptu sports jersey or serve as an emergency tourniquet or leak stopper.

GUYS' LIST ■

Most stylish guys for every modern style

One way to get a feel for fashion is to look at the guys who have perfected a certain look. A few model dressers on modern styles:

ALT SLOB *30 Rock*'s Judah Friedlander, in his uniform of ring-neck tees, baggy jeans, and bad-hair-covering hats, makes a statement with cleverly obscure phrases on his tee or lid, and standout sunglasses.

BLACK TIE Check out George Clooney at the Oscars: no bolo, no Nehru, no glitter. Clooney cops Cary Grant's Hollywood silhouettes and the Rat Pack macho edge, but never looks retro, only classic and smashing.

BUSINESS CASUAL Ever notice that Brad Pitt can wear a suit to a premiere or the beach and always look suave? That's because he wears his mostly solid suits snug, with fitted jackets and flat-front pants so that he's wearing the suit; it's not wearing him.

25 **How many pairs of jeans do I need?**

There are so many kinds of jeans, it's difficult at times to know what constitutes a guy's basic complement. Without question, you'll need a pair of classic prewashed or indigo boot-cut jeans that rides at your hip bones (no high-waisted elastic). If the classic cut's seam cleaves your glutes apart, you may want to try relaxed or loose-fit jeans. This timeless, basic look gives you maximum flexibility to wear jeans to

the office, out on a date, or lounging at home, and will stay in fashion

BUSINESS FORMAL Whatever you think of his politics, Barack Obama has reinstated an understated, simply tailored style to the office, with dark colors and white shirts paired with a bright, solid tie.

EVENING CHIC Ryan Seacrest's gig as *American Idol* emcee has made him such a fixture that you hardly notice what he's wearing—which is precisely why his laid-back jeans-and-jacket style is so brilliant.

PREPPY The Ivy League boys of Vampire Weekend spin traditional prep style forward, dressing up rugby shirts, striped dress shirts, cords, and Polo polos with white shoes over pink socks. Think classic—a chunky striped muffler like one of those toffs on *Gossip Girl*—paired with something offbeat or slightly ethnic.

ROCKER Pete Wentz of Fallout Boy bumps up Goth's mordant look to a sleek style. He layers hoodies over at least two shirts, with scarves on top. Below, it's stuck-to-skin jeans, in black or gray. A raggedly layered haircut finishes off the look.

URBAN Kanye West carries forward the fashion DNA of early rappers in geeky vests, cardigans, and slightly too-formal V-necks, but he's careful to combine his bow ties and argyle with sneakers, jean jackets, and ethnic scarves.

long enough for the denim to reach its ideal cottony softness and highly personalized fade.

Once you have the standard jeans, branch out into something fashionable—jeans that come prefaded or a pair of slightly dressier dark jeans. Even though fashion is the point, keep the effects to a minimum: nothing goes out of fashion faster than jeans with doodads. Remember that you'll need a belt that matches the jeans. A chunky cut demands a wide one; a rust-colored wash requires a strap of brown leather.

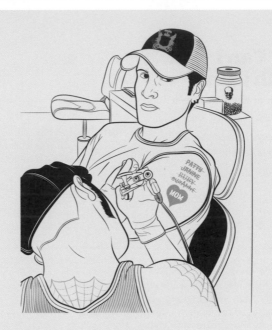

EXPERT WITNESS

26 HOW DO I PICK A TATTOO?

CHRIS NUÑEZ
co-owner, Love Hate Tattoos, Miami, Florida

"Don't try to clone what you see on TV or what some celebrity has, when it's you who's going to wear the design. Do the research until you're sure about what you're looking for: what style and what subject matter. Then find the best artist for that style, who'll translate and make it fit. Keep it clean and classic. Don't put too much detail in a small area, or mix genres—dragons with roses with dates and someone's name on top of it. You want a nice, neat package, not ten different tattoos in one spot. Then find an artist who'll translate your idea and make it fit."

27 Can I wear dress shoes with jeans?

Denim is like ketchup—it's hard to find anything that it doesn't go with. The best dress footwear for jeans is a pair of lace-up ankle boots (see page 23), but any oxford or loafer is a good companion. A faded pair of jeans and wing tips, especially with a natty cardigan buttoned up under a tweed jacket, is a classic look for fall.

28 When should I wear a tuxedo?

Anytime you get an invitation that reads "black tie" or "formal attire"— a wedding, a debutante ball, or the Academy Awards—you need to throw on a tux. If you want to get away with a black suit, make sure it's very crisp and chic, and add a silver-gray or deep purple tie on a white or light colored shirt.

29 Should I buy or rent?

Unless your job includes attending charity balls, a new tux is a difficult expense to justify. Even amortizing the cost of a new tux over renting seven or eight times in a decade presumes that you'll be able to fit into a tux you bought at age twenty-one, say, when you are creeping into middle age.

It's precisely this dynamic of formal wear, however, that populates vintage stores and hospital thrift shops with lightly used tuxedos cut for younger men's builds. Snap up a cast-off tux for cheap and have it tailored to your dimensions, and you'll always be prepared for a swanky affair, plus you'll look like a (inherited) million bucks.

30 **How do I accessorize a tux?**

Tuxedo shirts should be white, with simple pleats—no frilly ruffles—or plain front with a piqué texture, and fastened with shirt studs and cuff links instead of buttons. The patent-leather pump is the classic tuxedo shoe, but a black plain- or cap-toe oxford shoe is the perfect

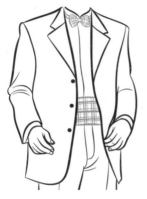

accompaniment.

Tuxedos have gotten closer to suits in style and cut in recent years, with regular neckties, ribbon ties, and even bolos substituting for the traditional bow tie. Use common sense as to whether the venue and the host will welcome deviations from custom. No matter what you have at your collar, never use a clip-on anything. (See page 145 to learn how to tie a bow tie.)

31 **Which way is up on my cummerbund?**

The open end of the pleats in the cummerbund always face upward—a rule you can remember by noting the reputed origin of the cummerbund as a crumb catcher designed to protect one's clothes at dinner.

32 Can I give my tux a personal touch?

Resist the urge to don alternate colors—blue or maroon or silver-gray jobs—that make you look like you're a refugee from a wedding band. The beauty of formal wear is precisely its conformity, by which you submit your individual importance to the significance of the event. You may, however, subtly give your tux some verve by wearing a dis-

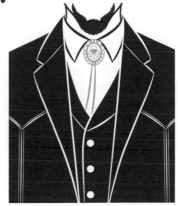

tinctive cummerbund and matching tie. Guys with Scots heritage for whom the kilt is too highland-heavy can wear a tartan plaid tie and cummerbund. Paisleys, moiré, and other patterns are also acceptable, as are colors like scarlet, midnight blue, or pink.

If you're in a wedding party, however, check with the groom or bride before you break the seamless black line.

33 **How much cologne should I use?**

You don't want to be that guy who everyone can smell coming. A spray on either side of your neck, dabbed with your wrists, is plenty for a normal day. To smell good when you go out at night, spray twice on your neck [a], and once a foot or so from your shirtfront [b], and walk into the cloud [c]. Never wear a scent to a job interview or on a first date, when it might compete with the woman's perfume.

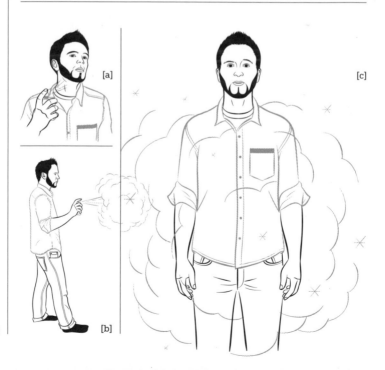

[a]

[b]

[c]

34 HOW DO I BEHAVE IN A RESTAURANT?

STEPHEN DUBLANACA
author of the book and the blog *Waiter Rant*

"Young men have such a terrible reputation for rudeness and unruliness in restaurants that there's a good chance you'll be treated as guilty—given a bad table at the back or ignored until you leave—before you sit down. Your fellow guys hit on women at other tables, try to get served alcohol when they are underage. They unbutton their pants when they get too full. Remember, a restaurant is a public place, but private property. You should be on your best behavior.

"Observing a few rules of etiquette will make it look like you know what you're doing. When you're being seated, follow the hostess or maître d' to the table. If you're the host, the youngest in your party, or the only male, allow others to precede you. When you get to your table, stand until the women or your elders are seated. Be sure to offer others a seat facing the rest of the room, which is the most comfortable view and keeps you from gazing over their shoulder for the whole meal. When you're ready to order, put your menu beside your plate, closed.

"Your waiter is there to help you have a good experience. Thank him or her, and your water server or busboy, each time you are served. When flagging any server down for a request, a simple 'excuse me' works; don't snap or call anyone 'waiter.' And keep your pants buttoned."

1
2
3
4
5
6

THE SOCIAL ANIMAL

35 **When should I shake hands?**

All introductions, from the most formal to the most casual, should include a handshake, and most random encounters can be celebrated with a handshake as well. When you greet a friend in company, shake with everyone in the group, whether you're acquainted or not, and introduce yourself by your name. A one-handed shake lasting no longer than it takes to say "How do you do?" fills the bill. Two-handed shaking is for diplomats or CEOs who've signed a major pact. Pumping the guy's hand relentlessly is for lonely uncles.

In some situations, the "bro' hug" has replaced handshaking among friends, male and female. A hug isn't always appropriate, however; offer your hand to a friend in case he or she wants to stop there; if all's okay, the handshake can still elide into an embrace. A guy-to-guy hug can be a full bear hug or a modified chest bump, with a momentary one-armed clasp, but with women keep it gentle and brief.

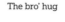
The bro' hug

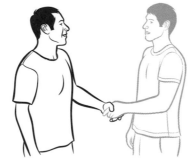
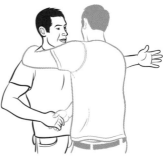

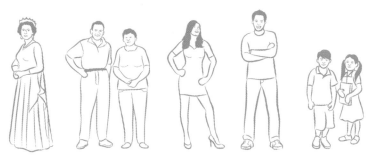

36 **What is the etiquette for making introductions?**

Esteemed, elderly, and female people (in that order) have the honor of being mentioned first, though the male, younger, or less significant person is the one actually being introduced. "Grandmom, this is my friend Sal," for example, or "Your Majesty, let me introduce my grandmother, Mrs. Smith." When a crowd of folks is being introduced, the same hierarchy applies: "Grandmom, here are Judy, Bob, and Dave," but you may want to break people into groups of respect. For instance, "Grandmom, please meet my boss, Mr. Smith. And these are my colleagues Bob and Dave." In formal situations, it's customary for the introducer to stand to one side of the two new acquaintances and extend a hand toward the person being introduced.

37 **When should I stand up to greet someone?**

Always stand for a woman, a person of an older generation, and anyone else you're going to be shaking hands with, even casually.

There are circumstances when a guy doesn't have to stand up to greet, meet, or acknowledge the presence of another person—when you're introduced to a peer on a crowded, moving bus, say, and definitely when a pal walks into the room where you're loafing on a sofa. In other cases, however, a guy shaking from a seated position usually looks either arrogant or feminine.

38 **What about the social kiss?**

It's better to let a woman offer her cheek rather than assume she'll welcome a kiss. If she does, press a small area of your cheek lightly against her cheekbone, taking care not to smudge any makeup. You needn't make contact with your lips, but be sure to graze the other person's cheek: a complete whiff, known as an "air kiss," comes off as fake and precious.

Social kissing is a more developed art in Europe and Latin America. Be prepared for European visitors to kiss more ardently, on both cheeks—in some countries, close friendship dictates three kisses, alternating cheeks—and men often kiss men as readily as they do women. In business situations Stateside, however, kisses are generally considered unprofessional, even between close friends and opposite sexes. Anytime you prefer not to be kissed, gently stiffen your arm as you shake hands to maintain your distance and subtly step back. The would-be kisser should get the hint.

39 How do I take someone out for an important meal?

Your first order of business is to choose the right restaurant, which means one that suits both your purpose and your guest's needs. Don't try to have a business conversation while jumping up constantly to hit a buffet, and don't take a vegetarian to a steak house. A late reservation isn't suitable for an elderly person or a friend with young children.

If possible, pick a restaurant you've eaten in before and like, and where you know the menu and the waitstaff. If you chose a new place, drop by earlier in the day or, better yet, a few days before, around the time of your reservation. Familiarize yourself with the menu, request a particular table, even chat with a waiter. If it's the day of your reservation, ask what the specials are (and how much they cost). When you show up later with your boss or hot date, you'll have your mind on the matters at hand.

40 What is considered a proper tip?

Tip between 15 and 20 percent of your total check. Twenty has become the standard for decent-to-above-average service; don't hesitate to give your waitperson a bonus on top of that for anything above and beyond the call of duty. If you're disappointed with the service—and not the quality of the meal, which is the chef's responsibility—you should still leave 15 percent. In many restaurants, the waitstaff splits their tips with the bartender or the busboy, neither of whom should be punished for a waiter's sins. Cheapness can backfire: your date may take a peek at how much you've tipped.

41 **How do I cure myself of being a wallflower?**

A crowd at a party or a business gathering can feel overwhelming. Set yourself the goal of getting to know one person better. Get his or her story: at the workplace, how did she come to work there? How's the commute? At a party, ask how a nearby guest knows the host or hostess. Throw the focus on someone else, and your own self-consciousness will fade away.

42 **What do I say to make small talk?**

Think of conversation as a team sport, not a solo performance. Be interested instead in what others are saying. Ask a pertinent question—"What did you mean when you said . . ." or "How was that different from what you expected"— to draw people out. Once he or she starts talking, it will likely remind you

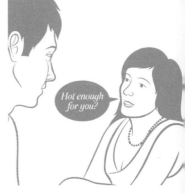

Hot enough for you?

of experiences you've had that illustrate what your interlocutor is saying. No story is so fascinating as one that backs up their point.

43 **To friend or not to friend?**

The point of social networking is not intimacy, nor should you consider all your online friends your true ones. So while it doesn't make sense to friend up with someone you've never heard of, in general apply an open-door policy. If you are uncomfortable granting them a view into your inner circle, use privacy settings, the "hide" feature, and other restrictions on who can post to your page to deal with the hassles of having a large body of online associates.

44 **How do I hang out with gay friends on their turf?**

Accompanying gay friends to a gay bar or other mostly gay gathering can be a little unnerving for a straight guy. You're suddenly the odd man out, and being checked out—both of which can make a guy (who's used to doing the checking out) very self-conscious. No need to sweat. Gay men are used to detecting when another man is available and interested. Though your presence on gay turf might momentarily confuse the issue, be yourself and the room will soon pick up on your heterosexuality. If you do get an overt invitation, calmly say that you're with friends and move along—if your friends don't notice and inform him of your status first. Meantime, take the rare chance to appreciate what it feels like to be in the sexual minority—which is how your gay friends feel most of the time.

1
2
3
4
5
6

45 How do I order personal stationery?

Antiquated as it may seem, stationery made by a print shop with your name atop it and a matching envelope makes an impression—namely that your sentiments are worthy of a proper setting. For less than $100, you can order a run of personalized eight-by-five-inch half-sheet notepads with matching envelopes that will last you forever. (You may want to leave your address off the envelopes so you can still use them as you move residences.)

Ordering stationery requires three basic decisions—about paper stock, paper color, and a fitting typeface. Use at least a twenty-four-pound bond paper; anything lighter feels flimsy. Texture is a matter of taste: linen's light crosshatch, laid paper's horizontal pattern, and a smooth surface are equally appropriate. Color is a fun field to play in, but if you expect to use your stationery mostly for formal correspondence, stick to white, cream, gray, or light blue. You have more freedom with typefaces, especially now that computers set the font. Serifs—curlicues at the bottoms and tops of individual letters—are generally more formal, while sans serif fonts (like this one) project a modern mind-set.

A classic monogram is fine as a heading, but creativity is entirely welcome. If you're a skilled draftsman, by all means design your own, or invite a talented friend to do so. You may also want to order a second set of half sheets—for second and third pages of a letter with your initials tucked discreetly in a corner.

46 What's the best way to socialize with a recovering addict?

To start, it depends on how long they've been sober. If they are beyond the initial stages of risk—anywhere from six months to a year—socialize with them as you would with anyone else, especially if the night involves drinking on the lighter side—a glass of wine at dinner, a couple of beers with TV. Being overly conscious of their choice not to partake can sometimes be more annoying than considerate. And excluding them from plans—or at least an invitation—to go out can end friendships.

If the event involves more heavy drinking, like a pub crawl or a frat party, it's probably a good idea to let the sober person know that "Some of us—okay, all of us—are probably going to get really hammered." Some sober people will still come along. Others find being around people slurring and out of control annoying, and will take a pass.

But don't just abandon a friend who no longer participates in bar culture. Make an effort to work in some sober activities, like movies, eating out, nature walks, or bowling.

47 **Should a modern guy hold open doors?**

Some younger women take umbrage at gestures that imply they are weak: women, they object, are as capable as any guy. True enough, but the act of holding a door has little to do with physical strength. The motive is consideration, meaning you should hold a door for anyone, elderly ladies as well as your buffed pal who could rip the door from its hinges.

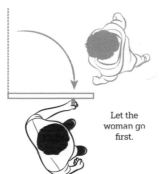
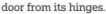

Let the woman go first.

You needn't race ahead to pull a door open and pose like Sir Galahad. A swift last step will get you there ahead of your walking partner. Nonchalantly swing it open and let the other person proceed. (The exception is a revolving door, which you enter first to get the door started.)

48 **What's the proper procedure at the urinals?**

When you have a choice, leave one or two urinals between you and anyone else answering nature's call. If the only free spot is next to a fellow urinator, act naturally. You are not required to stare ostentatiously at the ceiling. Keep your eyes up and front, don't moan or spit or otherwise disturb anyone's peace, even if it means suspending your conversation with your buddy across the room.

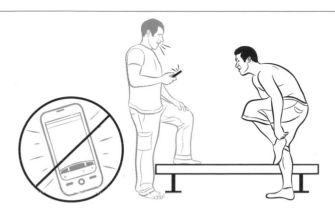

49 **What's proper locker-room etiquette?**

It's not just you: nobody is particularly comfortable stripping down and suiting up in the gym locker room, especially near the guy who flaunts his business like a porn star. For your sake and everyone else's, wear a towel when walking to and from the shower and while engaging in conversation. Respect other guys' privacy, keeping at a comfortable distance and casually finding another place to look while they are dressing. Don't wield your phone, especially in a way that suggests your camera could be recording. A lot of guys, clad or not, go to the gym for a little sanctuary, away from their hectic days. Be conscious of how much noise you're making, and if a guy doesn't seem interested in conversation, let him be. Once dressed, look around to check the condition of your area and wipe up any water or other mess you've left behind.

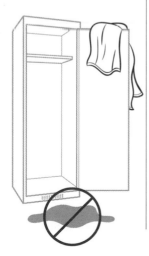

50 **When do I need to bring a gift to someone's house?**

Gifts are for special occasions—when you're a weekend guest, when you show up to see someone's new baby, or when your host or hostess has recently celebrated a birthday or anniversary. The gift should be somehow relevant: a board game for a weekend stay, baby clothing for the new arrival, and so on.

When invited to a casual house party, especially a dinner party, always ask if there's anything you can bring. If the host doesn't specify, a bottle of wine is always appreciated regardless (unless your guest is sober—take flowers instead), as is a small second dessert, like a pie, cookies, or fancy candies.

51 **How do I write a letter?**

You aren't likely to put pen to paper these days unless you have momentous news or something special to say. The formality of a handwritten letter can make writing it tough.

You've put the date at the top, the salutation ("Dear Mom," or "Hey Dude"), and then, even if you're bursting with news, it can be difficult to know where to begin. The classic opening to a friendly letter is a conversational greeting, but with so many more immediate forms of communicating, and the heightened expectations prompted by a letter's arrival these days, "How are you?" is a waste of words. Instead, set the scene for your announcement: where you are writing from ("My trip to Argentina has been amazing . . ."), or how you are feeling ("I never thought I'd write this letter . . .").

After this brief drumroll, get right to your big news. The next few paragraphs should offer a rationale for your decision, or, if the matter isn't especially controversial, some play-by-play on how it came to pass. You may want to write out this section of your letter on scrap paper before committing it to your card or stationery—as the old saying goes, "How do I know what I want to say before I've said it?" A draft prevents cross-outs and rewrites.

Another paragraph or so looking forward—next steps, further obstacles, or incidental details—brings you to a line of conclusion, wishing your reader well, and sign-off. Traditional sign-offs for those close to you, besides a simple "love," are "best wishes," "fondly," or the standard "yours."

Of course, you don't have to have anything important to say. A personal letter is always welcome, and the older the person you are contacting, the more appropriate paper feels. In these cases, the above format still stands: your news may just be more run-of-the-mill, and your justifications more whimsical.

52 How do I write a thank-you note?

Paper is the gold standard when saying thank you. It's old-fashioned, but the thanks can't be doubted when it comes via a handwritten, hand-stamped piece of mail. Put pen to paper for a weekend at someone's house; a birthday, wedding, or anniversary gift; a lunch hosted by someone of an elder generation; or a floral arrangement sent to your relative's funeral. The contents of the note are less important than the gesture, so don't chew your pencil over what to say. "Thanks again for . . ." or "Just a note to thank you for . . ." is a perfectly acceptable beginning, to be followed with "Great to see you" or "Let's do it at my place next time." If you can work in a personal touch, do so—for instance, after a weekend getaway, a mention of your favorite moment or a hope that the host is resting up after that strenuous volleyball game is icing on the cake.

An e-mail or a quick phone call is fine to say thanks for a casual dinner or brunch at a friend's house or tickets to a ball game, as long as the giver is a friend; if your boss or a friend of your parents' hosted you, a note will perk up everyone involved.

Thanks for gifts are a separate category. As a rule, if a gift is opened in front of the gifter, and you thank them appropriately, you don't need to send a note. Then again, written thanks are *never* wasted.

53 Should I carry a calling card?

The personal card is making a comeback lately, perhaps by dint of the sheer amount of information that clings to us these days—work and personal e-mail addresses, cell and landline numbers, IM handles, and snail-mail address.

If you're self-employed, you definitely want to carry a personal calling card. Traditionally your name alone goes in the center of a personal card—no need to assign yourself a cutesy title like "Human Being." But if you're listing all your contact data, you'll want your name to stand out: put it on the left and the laundry list of ways to reach you below. Any custom printing shop—and an increasing number of Web outlets—can help you with a design, including graphic elements to make the card stand out.

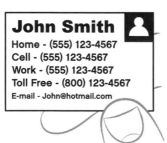

John Smith
Home - (555) 123-4567
Cell - (555) 123-4567
Work - (555) 123-4567
Toll Free - (800) 123-4567
E-mail - John@hotmail.com

If your employer furnishes you with a business card, you still may want to have personal cards made. A personal card is less formal and can be useful if you don't want to give someone your business phone and e-mail address. In a pinch, you can give a special someone the inside dope by writing your personal information on the back of your business card.

GUYS' LIST

The two best rock guitarists you've never heard of

1 **TOMMY BOLIN** His fame came as the guy who replaced other greats when they left their bands, but among guitar insiders Bolin is regarded as a major force in the fusion movement, with some putting him above Jeff Beck in that movement's pantheon. His last album, *Private Eyes,* recorded shortly before Bolin died of drug and alcohol abuse, is the one many fans treasure most.

2 **LES DUDEK** A teen prodigy, Dudek has played for artists as diverse as Steve Miller, Boz Scaggs, Stevie Nicks, and Cher (whom he dated). He's best known for helping Allman's lead guitarist Dickey Betts finish some of the tunes on *Brothers and Sisters* after Duane Allman died, and he shares a writing credit on "Jessica." His peak came on his first three solo albums, which meld southern rock and fusion.

1
2
3
4
5
6

THE THINGS WE DO FOR BUDS

54 **What should I wear to a wedding?**

Unless the invitation calls for black tie (or Wiccan robes), you can assume a wedding is business formal, even if the vows are to be taken outdoors. A plain navy or dark gray suit is appropriate morning, noon, or night; for summer nuptials planned for morning or early afternoon (including the reception), a tan or blue khaki suit is more than acceptable; white, whether in pants, jacket, or an ensemble, is for the bride, and not for you.

55 **What are a best man's responsibilities?**

Your chief task, besides handing the groom the ring when he turns for it, is to throw a bachelor party. Traditional activities center around naked women, avid drinking, and sexual pranks, but as the sight of a naked woman is hardly a rare treat for a guy these days—and as we invest more time and money in our weddings—the strip-club bachelor party is increasingly being abandoned for alternative bonding experiences, like extreme sports events or weekend getaways. Have a conversation with the groom to gauge what level of risky business he's up for. You can surprise him with a bit of random bawdiness without making the entire enterprise about illicit sex.

If you don't live close to the groom, enlist his friends or brothers to help with the arrangements. Plan the romp as close to the wedding

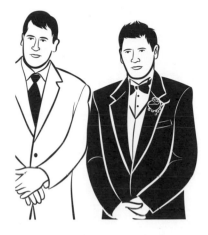

Do whatever it takes to make the groom comfortable.

as you can manage, but not for the night before: the guy wants to be present and cogent for the most important day of his young life.

Once you're on-scene, you're the groom's right-hand man, helping him to make sure that all's running smoothly, from picking up stray arrivals at the airport to accompanying his unattended aunt into the rehearsal dinner to laughing at his nervous jokes and making sure his tie is straight.

Expect to say a few words at the rehearsal dinner, but your star turn comes at the reception, where your toast is, for many guests, the keynote speech. Try not to be too serious, or too ribald—the groom's grandmother-in-law doesn't mind references to youthful high jinks, but she doesn't want to hear the details. The point is how your boy's life changed when he met his beloved, and how happy you are for both of them. Start with a funny story—perhaps the moment you realized his goose was cooked, or about a girlfriend sufficiently lost in the past (like the first grade)—then move on. Offer some philosophy of life from your still tender perspective, acknowledge the friends who have come a long way or who go a long way back, and finish up with a toast to the happy couple.

56 What do I do if I can't attend a friend's wedding?

Send a letter explaining how disappointed you are to miss your pal's big day, and send or personally deliver a gift anytime up to a year after the wedding. As soon as you have the chance, take him and his bride out to dinner and demand that they show you pictures and tell you all about the day.

57 How do I attend an unfamiliar religious ceremony?

Dress should be formal, with shoes shined and a close shave—the pal who invited you is going to be seeing you through the eyes of the most aged relative on the scene. Also wear a decent pair of socks, since in places like Hindu temples, shoes are removed at the door. As long as you're not directly involved in any of the proceedings, visiting a friend's house of worship usually demands more patience than anything else. Your job is to bear it with good humor mixed with the appropriate dose of solemnity. Be open, and you may even enjoy it.

58 What gift should I give for a religious ceremony I'm unfamiliar with?

If you're not sure what kind of religious paraphernalia goes with the rite in question, something age-appropriate will do: a silver rattle, baby spoon, or a baby dining set for a baby's baptism; for a coming-of-age ceremony, like a bar mitzvah or a confirmation, a check or cash in an envelope for the young person is almost always appropriate.

No matter the religion, for a wedding, give a household item geared toward the couple's life together. Remember this is the one chance for them to collect useful gifts, like kitchen tools and decorative platters, that no one will ever give them again.

59 Should I attend the wake or the funeral?

You should always go to all related events when someone close to you dies. When it's the relative of a friend, or someone you don't know well, there's always the awkward question of which events to attend.

You should always feel comfortable attending a memorial service, which is designed for anyone who wants to pay his or her respects. Don't hesitate to attend a wake. Call the funeral home to ascertain the hours the event begins and ends. Wear a tie and a jacket. A member of the family will often greet you at the door, giving you the opportunity to offer your condolences. "I'm sorry for your loss" is simple enough. Sign the guest book. Go to the casket (immediately if no one greets you) and briefly pay your respects to the body; a kneeler is usually provided, but don't feel you have to kneel. Don't be shy about comforting people with words, a handshake, or a hug. After half an hour or so of subdued chatting, you're free to go.

The closer you are to the family of the dead person, the more likely it is that you'll be expected to go to the funeral (the most common religious service followed by the burial) or visit a religious Jewish family at home as they sit shivah (a traditional seven-day mourning period). Your presence there won't be unwelcome—empty funerals are depressing—and if you admired the deceased or feel like showing respect for those grieving, you should go.

Even if you attend the service, the trip to the cemetery is a must-do only for those in the family and very close friends.

60 How do I stop a friend from trying to sell me his newfound religion?

Your friend believes that he has just discovered something so wonderful that he wants you to have it, too. In his mind, he's trying to give you a great gift—the gift of his religion. The difficult part is that you

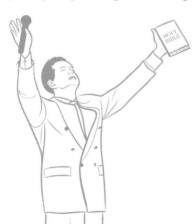

don't really want what he has. It doesn't fit you, you don't like the design or designer, or you already have one and you prefer yours. The only way to stop your friend is to let him know that while it may be perfect for him, you don't want it for you. If he really won't leave you alone after you have been direct, stop hanging out until your pal calms down a bit, as most converts eventually do.

61 **How do I get rid of an annoying friend?**

An old friend will know when he's done you wrong and won't need any explaining, but you may want to spell out your hurt or disagreement for your own sake. If you're never going to talk to him again, that's a long time to have something on your chest.

More common is the need to blow off someone who has adopted you as his best pal when you don't have much in common. Think in terms of time management. Tell your aspiring buddy that you need to pay more attention to work and are cutting down on hanging out. If he doesn't take the hint, you may have to get more explicit, but at least you gave him the chance to go away with his dignity.

62 **How do I tell my friend I'm gay?**

Don't dismiss the idea that your friend already knows, or suspects. He may already be pondering why you haven't had a girlfriend in a while, or why you've been hanging out with guys he's never met. Ask mutual friends how much he knows already.

Whether he has a clue or not, don't let your anxiety or need for sudden clarity (like your boyfriend's demands to be recognized as such) drive you to make a big announcement in a way that it leaves your friend no room to process the information. Let him know you've been questioning your status. Explain that your new friends are gay (if they're out), and that you've been doing some thinking. Educate him about stereotypes of gay life as a way of guiding his reaction.

1
2
3
4
5
6

If he doesn't take it well, remember that coming out is about you, and not him. If he's a good enough friend, he'll come around to it; if not, it's his loss.

Once he's used to the idea, inject some humor into the situation. Remind him that he's got one less competitor for the chicks, or that, gay or no, you can still whip him on the basketball court. And remember to be diplomatic when he asks if you have ever been attracted to him (because unless he's read the next entry already, he might ask).

63 What do I say when a friend comes out to me?

Your pal has probably put a lot of thought into how to tell you he's gay, and he may have weathered some anxiety over the best time and way to do so. Your first move should be to thank him for telling you, as it means he values your friendship. Be honest about your feelings—he'll be able to tell if you're covering up—but remember that his decision to come out is a milestone for him, not for you. Keep your cool and ask how he's dealing—what it means for his life and who else he's told. You'll have plenty of time later to process what your pal's love life means for you. And don't ask him if he finds you attractive. It only makes the situation more awkward.

2

Necessities

We guys have needs that occupy most of our waking thoughts: work, friends, sex, this weekend's dose of harmless destruction. Then there are the hassles we can't get along without: a place to crash, the wheels we're driving until we get our dream ride, a sensible place for our money. Organized thinking about these issues is a hassle in itself, but once done, clears your mind for pursing more immediate goals. ▶

HOME ECONOMICS

64 **How do I establish a realistic budget?**

There's no mystery—and no mercy—to writing up a budget. To save yourself a lot of misery, be honest with yourself in accounting for your expenses, including miscellanies like beer, music downloads, and gifts for the significant other. These are legitimate and inevitable outflows for a guy. Ignore or discount them, and your budget will be shot full of holes every month.

Be sure to anticipate intermittent bills as well. Once you've toted up your weekly and monthly spending, go back a year or so in your bank statements, financial software, or checkbook looking for dental bills, car repairs, and vacations. Add up what you spent on these items and divide by twelve (months) to come up with their monthly average, and count them into your budget.

It's perfectly possible that, having subtracted your actual expenses from your take-home pay, you'll have a shortfall. This is an opportunity to examine your priorities. Remember, don't balance your budget on the back of foregoing temptations, like that second glass of wine with dinner. Instead, look to savings you can't reverse at a moment's notice: canceling services you don't use—your home internet if you can poach from others, your cable if you can rent DVDs of your favorite shows instead, and your landline if you bother with one. Suspend your gym membership for the summer, when you can easily get your exercise outdoors.

65 Should I file my own tax return?

It depends on how you make your money and how much you make. The world is simple for guys who are on a salary, with taxes taken out, and make less than $100,000 per annum. Each year, as tax season rolls around, your employer sends a W-2 form informing you how much the company told the IRS it paid you and how much it has already sent to the Feds for safekeeping. Banks, mutual funds, and anyone else who paid out interest or dividends send similar forms. You transfer the data from the W-2 and other forms onto another form called a 1040EZ (or an equally simple form, the 1040A, if you have stock dividends to report as well as interest income). You can also use these forms to list income from gambling, tips, or unemployment benefits. The combined amount is your gross income.

Next, subtract your personal exemption and your standard deduction—two gimme tax breaks the government allows you for the cost of being you. The result is your taxable income. Now you look up the tax on that amount on a chart provided in the instruction booklet or online. If what the government withheld is more than you owe, you get a refund; less than that, and you owe. Once you're done, you have to complete another very similar return for the state you live in.

The good news is that you can file online. If you can order a book on Amazon, you can get through the 1040EZ.

The forms multiply as your sources and amount of income multiply. If you made more than $100,000 in taxable income or didn't work for a company in the traditional way, you have to use the grown-up 1040 form, which comes with a lot more paperwork. Independent contractors of any kind—nonsalaried construction workers and pool boys, freelancers of all kinds, or a guy with his own ice-cream truck—file a Schedule C, declaring income (or loss) from a small business. Schedules B and D register income from dividends and capital gains (what you make when you sell investments for a profit) respectively. This all constitutes your gross income.

Now you take your personal exemption and deductions (the standard, or—if you can beat it with deductions for business outlays, charitable contributions, and other expenses—Schedule A) and subtract from your gross income, and figure the tax on what's left.

If your life is complicated enough to need the 1040 form, it's worth going to see a professional tax preparer at least once to get a tax checkup, the way you would a checkup from a doctor. You may be eligible for tax exemptions that you are unaware of, or you may be overlooking deductions. Once the accountant has established a model for you, you're set until your financial picture changes and you need a new checkup.

66 **Can I lessen the tax bite on my paycheck?**

The W-4 form you fill out your first day at work helps determine how much of your salary your employer withholds from your paycheck and forwards to the IRS, but the information is not legally binding. If you want to keep more of your money now rather than wait for a refund come April 15, increase the number of dependents you claim on the W-4, adding one or two. Don't go overboard, or you'll end up paying a bundle of tax when you file your return plus a fine for underwithholding. But there's nothing illegal about right-sizing your withholding by using the dependents box.

67 How do I balance my checking account?

Whether or not you actually write checks, that check register they gave you when you opened your account is a useful way to keep track of your expenditures and deposits. About once a week, enter every stray ATM slip and debit receipt and check you've written into your checkbook register and bring down the numbers so you know how much you think you have. The more complete your register, the faster and less stressful it will be to justify the numbers with your bank. You can use financial software like Quicken to do this, too.

Go to your bank's Web site. Your recent transactions for each account will be listed, probably in reverse-date order. Check off every transaction that both you and your bank have recorded. Add transactions that the bank recorded that you forgot. Subtract again in your checkbook.

On your online statement, the bank will show your balance. Subtract from this outstanding checks and debit-card purchases that haven't shown up in your account yet. The result should be the balance you show in your checkbook, or close to it. Don't kill yourself trying to justify a few dollars' discrepancy. Note any small difference as a debit or a credit in order to match the bank's number and move on. If the difference is significant, do the math again. If it persists after subtracting again, you may want to contact your bank.

68 How should I pay my bills?

The world of personal finance has gone online, and there is no reason you should not use online banking when it is convenient and safe.

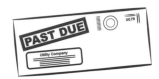

Financial software or your bank's Web site will pay your monthly bills automatically the moment they are due, allowing bill payers to "set it and forget it." In truth, relegating your financial life to computers only saves you the paperwork: you should still check in frequently to make sure you're keeping up with increases in your bills, mistaken overcharges, and to make sure that you've got enough income to cover your outflow.

In order to prevent overdrafts, and make a little hay out of your expenses, consider disconnecting your bills from your checking account and putting all your monthly expenditures on a credit card with a decent rewards program that pays in air miles or vacation points. With a high enough spending limit, you'll never "bounce" a payment to a creditor, and every annoying bill comes with a bonus. Just be sure to pay off your credit card balance in full every month to avoid finance charges.

69 **How should I reduce my credit-card balances?**

It pays—literally—to pay off your credit card balance in full every month. Living within your means provides the kind of freedom that a life based on credit won't, since debt will follow you for years to come.

But hey, things come up, and if you do end up owing some money, here's what you can do to get rid of it.

First, collect all of your cards and put them away. Give them to a trusted relative, put them in a container of water and jam it in the freezer, or cut them up. That will slow, if not stop, you from using them.

Next, figure out what you owe. Find out what the minimum payment is on each balance, and what interest rate you're being charged. Now throw everything you have at the card with the smallest balance. Pay only the minimum on the others. Once the first card is paid off, proceed to the next-largest balance and do the same thing. Repeat until you're debt-free.

You'll be tempted by what seem like daily offers to transfer your debt to a new credit card with no interest on your existing balance. Take advantage of only those offers that have no transfer fees attached, and pay close attention to the rate you'll be charged once the introductory no-interest period expires—if you can't pay off the balance before the rate kicks in, you may end up paying more in the long run than you are now. More important, when your new card arrives, cancel your old one (this can take some doing, as most credit-card companies resist your initial demands to close your account), and never activate the new one. Otherwise, you'll just have another black hole into which to sink your dough.

70 **What can I do to make some extra cash?**

A fascination with bodily fluids causes some guys to think selling their blood or sperm is the coolest route to quick dough. Selling your plasma—the liquid your blood cells flow in—is the most profitable fluid-related gig, paying anywhere from ten to sixty dollars, depending on shortages and your location. Plasma is also the fastest. The only instant

1
2
3
4
5
6

gratification you'll get from sperm sales is the kind you'll be giving yourself: in general, sperm banks test and retest your goods over the course of weeks and months, and anyway the pay is not life-changing.

Better plans for fast, low-skill cash are tip-generating gigs like bartending or waiting tables for a caterer or—if you're determined to bring your manhood into it—posing nude for art classes.

71 **How do I save money?**

Saving money is easiest if you never see it. Sign up for automatic deposit, and divide your paycheck between your checking account and a savings, money-market, or mutual-fund account. Now pretend that the saved portion of the money doesn't exist. As it accrues interest over time, it will add up.

Alternatively, segregate income from different sources. Let's say you do work for two major clients, or you moonlight. Try living on the larger check exclusively while you deep-six the other employer's check in your savings.

And don't forget the easiest way to save for the future—enroll in your company's 401(k) plan. A lot of companies will match what you put in, which is effectively additional untaxed salary—otherwise known as free money. You can't access it until you're ready to retire, but it will grow, with interest that the IRS won't touch until you begin to make withdrawals.

72 **How do I get into day trading?**

There's a common misconception that day trading is normal investing conducted at a fast pace. Day traders don't go by traditional indicators like P&E ratios. Day trades are driven by odd statistical patterns in how particular stocks rise and fall. All you need in order to make money—eventually—is a particular strategy that makes use of those patterns and the discipline to apply it, even when all hell is breaking loose. Otherwise, it helps to have some trading software, a robust Wi-Fi connection, and about $5,000 to open an account.

EXPERT WITNESS

73 WHERE SHOULD I PUT MY RETIREMENT FUND?

GEORGE MANNES
senior writer, *Money* magazine

"In addition to your 401(k), which is a free-money no-brainer if your company is matching your contributions (and recommended even if it's not), you probably want to get yourself a Roth IRA. The Roth is like a regular IRA (which stands for 'individual retirement account'), in that its money compounds tax-free—as it grows, dividends are reinvested, untaxed, as long as they remain in the account. In a regular IRA, however, you pay taxes on the money once you start withdrawing it—which you can start doing once you are 59.5 years old; in a Roth, you don't. What's the catch? The money you put into a Roth is after-tax money. But since most of you are probably in a lower tax bracket now, it's better to take the tax hit when you are young than later, when your tax rate is usually steeper."

74 **Which should I use: a debit card or cash?**

Experts who have studied the issue believe that paying cash inhibits spending, especially what the pros call collateral spending (like adding a candy bar onto your gas purchase). Handing over cash money, perhaps, carries more emotional weight than sliding a debit card through a reader, which doesn't even feel like you're spending. Even though a debit card keeps an automatic record of your transactions and doesn't create highly fritter-away-able small bills and coins, you're likely to save more if you carry cash for day-to-day transactions.

75 **Which stocks should I buy?**

The funny-talking baby on the Super Bowl commercials might have given you the impression that you can make a safe, rational killing on the stock market. In fact, most of us don't have the knowledge, time, or resources to bet on individual stocks. It's better to do okay with mutual funds than to try to score big with stocks.

If, however, you do buy stocks on your own account, pick a discount broker with a flat per-transaction charge and a minimum account balance you can live with. For long-term plays, many companies allow you to circumvent brokers altogether through their direct reinvestment programs. DRIPs, as they are known, aren't made for buying and selling quickly—you make a profit on an initial purchase of a number of shares and the company automatically invests any dividends in more shares for you. Over time, your account grows to a respectable number of shares.

76 Do I need a will if I don't really own anything?

A will is not about who gets your beloved collection of concert T-shirts. It's not even about your investments, since you can name a beneficiary when you do the paperwork for all your financial accounts. For a younger person, the best reason to write a will is to leave a living will that includes instructions about medical decisions in case you're incapacitated. Stating your wishes formally saves your relatives a bunch of hassles and heartache. While you're at it, you can declare, for the record, that your worldly effects should go to your parents, or your siblings. You don't have to pay a lawyer. Get a form from the Internet, have it notarized, and keep it with your passport in a place your family is sure to find it.

77 Should I rent or buy?

The sooner you get into the housing market, the more money you'll make. Unlike securities, real estate solves two problems at once. I have to pay to live somewhere, some guys figure, why not sock my investment money into something I own?

That's a good impulse, but you should know that renting is historically cheaper than buying: you're insulated against property-tax increases and the cost of repairs. Even counting the huge tax break you get as a home owner (the IRS lets you deduct the interest you pay on your mortgage, as well as your property taxes), home ownership comes up short.

This rule of thumb presumes, however, that every penny you save by renting will end up in some other investment. And that's not too likely.

So you should buy, right? Hold on. For a young guy, the balance tips toward renting. With what you're making right now, the mortgage-interest tax break may not amount to much actual cash. For another thing, younger people are mobile: more likely to be assigned out of state, more likely to move for romantic reasons or simply to change their minds about where they want to live.

And remember while you can always suspend payments to a stock fund if you decide to chuck it all and backpack across China, a mortgage payment is due every month until you pay it off or sell the house. Until you are ready to settle down for a while—five years is the rule—stay liquid.

78 How do I buy a house?

You've decided on a neighborhood you like: it's got homes you can afford, a commute you can handle, a restaurant with good burgers. You have some dough set aside. Now what?

▶ **SECURE A LOAN FIRST** Imagine you are selling your car. One buyer says he'll pay you now. Another offers more but has to see if his mom will lend him the money. Whom do you sell it to? The guy with the cash. For the same reason, you may win the bidding on a house if your financing is already in place. So don't even shop for a house without a letter of preapproval in hand. (Not prequalified, which is a nice vote of confidence, but not a guarantee of a loan.)

You don't have to get your cash from a local lender—out-of-town banks, which you can find online, may have better rates. (Your corner bank is going to administer your loan by a faceless computer anyway.) Apply for as much money as you think you can qualify for.

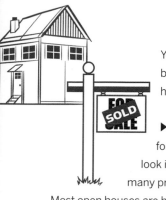

You don't have to borrow all of what you've been preapproved for, but when the bidding heats up, you'll want some headroom.

▶ **SHOP** Cruise your target neighborhood for "For Sale" signs, talk with agents, and look in the newspaper for open houses. Visit as many properties as you have time and patience for. Most open houses are held on weekends. If you can take a day off during the week before an advertised open house, you may beat the competition to a good buy. Be thorough, but don't second-guess yourself; if the first house you see looks like the one you've envisioned, pull the trigger.

Remember that, as nice as Realtors are, they represent the seller. You may want to seek out a buyer's agent—a licensed realty agent who is working for you.

▶ **MAKE AN OFFER** Once you've found a house, you need to come up with an opening bid. If the market is hot and there are multiple bidders, you may have to open with the asking price if you really want the house.

In a slower market, you have time to do some homework. Compare the asking prices of surrounding houses. On the Internet or at the local library, you'll find "comps": listings of recent home sales in the area and what the final price was. Apartment prices are usually calculated per square foot; houses are less tightly quantified.

Obviously, you want to start the bidding as low as you can, but don't insult the seller with an obvious lowball offer. A seller's agent can't tell you what everyone else is bidding, so elicit hints by asking, "How do you think that will be received?" Never bid twice in one conversation. If you hear your bid is insufficient, ask that the house not be sold without giving you a chance to bid again and retreat to study your next move.

▶ **RETAIN COUNSEL** You won! Before you go to contract and set up a date for a settlement or closing, where the checks will be written (mostly by you) and the deed handed over, you'll want a lawyer to walk you through the process.

79 **How do I buy a house in a neighborhood I can't afford?**

Look for a house in disrepair, which can sell at 5 to 20 percent below its neighbors—possibly enough to give you the leg up you need. Some repairs could be deal breakers—have the property inspected early on for serious structural problems, like a cracked foundation or unstable joists and beams, before you commit. But if the engineer gives a thumbs-up, jump in.

Some people observe that the cost of fixing up a handyman's special usually brings the eventual price of the house close to the area's standard anyway. Repair things in your own sweet time, and in the meantime you don't pay mortgage interest on their cost. (In fact, it's important to save all the receipts: when you sell, these costs often get added to your basis, reducing your profit on paper and thus decreasing the capital gains tax that you're liable for.)

80 **Should I buy a house from a relative?**

Let's say your parents or a favorite uncle and aunt are ready to get rid of a house and are willing to sell to you. It's great for you—you don't have to go through the pain of looking at houses and deciding which is right. It's great for them—your relative saves the percentage of the purchase price they'd pay a broker. Sounds like a bargain, right? Just make sure you think the idea all the way through before you just say yes. Awkward issues may come up when your familial relationship becomes a business one.

First, sit down with your relative to discuss how you will deal with the costs aside from the purchase price. You should pay for fees relating to the transfer of the deed—as you would if you were buying from a stranger, but other questions remain: Who pays for repairs that come to light during the process? Will you split the amount of a Realtor's commission between you, since this is normally factored into the sale price? Who pays for the lawyer to draw up a contract? What about court filing and clerk fees? Your parents, being your parents, may make generous concessions, but you don't want to live with their second thoughts the rest of your lives.

For this reason, it's important to have a licensed real-estate assessor come up with a market value for the place—an objective, professional opinion will save a lot of misgivings or recrimination later. (It may be wise to have each party have a separate estimate done and then split the difference to determine the purchase price.) After the purchase price is agreed upon, hire a single lawyer to close the deal for both sides.

1

2
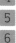
3
4
5
6

FEATHERING YOUR NEST

81 **What equipment do I need in the kitchen?**

Not every guy is going to be a master chef, but cooking—like any job—is easier with the right tools. Here's what you'll need:

▶ **TEN-INCH-DIAMETER CAST-IRON PAN** A versatile frying pan is perfect for eggs, bacon, pancakes, stir-fry, steak.

▶ **SET OF HEAVY-BOTTOMED POTS** To whip up a bowl of spaghetti, chili, steamed vegetables, or curry. (If you don't want to buy the whole set, pick out one that fits the serving size you'll be making.)

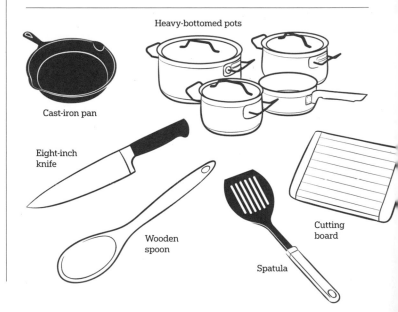

Heavy-bottomed pots

Cast-iron pan

Eight-inch knife

Wooden spoon

Spatula

Cutting board

▶ **WOODEN SPOON** Handy for stirring, tasting, serving.

▶ **SPATULA** Convenient for flipping, scraping, serving. If you have nonstick pans, pick a plastic one that won't scrape up the cookware's surface.

▶ **CUTTING BOARD** Necessary for food prep, serving. (A colorful plastic one doubles as a cheese platter and goes right in the dishwasher.)

▶**EIGHT-INCH KNIFE** Use for everything. You don't have to be on *Top Chef* to know that a chef's knife is his most important tool. Be prepared to pay a little extra for this item. Forged-steel knives have good balance and keep their edge nicely, so most cooks prefer them over stamped-steel ones.

82 **What should a guy stock in his kitchen?**

You'll never go hungry if you have the following items in healthy quantities:

▶ **BACON** Think of bacon as a condiment that tops off a sandwich (turkey, grilled cheese, or peanut butter), salad, or anything that needs a big hit of flavor. Simplify by cooking it in the microwave.

▶ **BEANS** The army has traditionally made beans a staple for the fighting man for a reason. Make that a few reasons: beans keep well,

1
2
3
4
5
6

cook up easily, and deliver high amounts of protein, fiber, and iron to keep you on your feet and punching. Kidney, pinto, black, great northern, or little white beans can all be added to salads or tossed with tuna or pasta. A can of lentil soup can be an instant pasta sauce.

▶ **HOT SAUCE** Does it really matter what you're eating, as long as it blows the lid off your mouth and leaves you in a postendorphin glow? The hot-sauce industry has exploded in recent years, with dozens of artisanal makers. So besides being a make-good for your bland cooking skills, hot sauce collecting can become your hobby.

▶ **OATMEAL** A cylinder of quick oats puts you within a few minutes' worth of microwaving a breakfast or snack that not only cleans the pipes and mitigates the effects of cholesterol but cheers you up. Have apples, raisins, and cinnamon nearby and add them about halfway through the box's prescribed zapping time. For the extra lazy, there's the instant version (in which case go with Irish steel-cut oats or you'll sacrifice too much taste).

▶ **OLIVE OIL** Tasty enough to eat raw—toss in a few flakes of basil or chili pepper and use it in place of butter—olive oil is the starting point for a hundred meals. Pour a few tablespoons into a warming pan, add a little chopped garlic, and contemplate what's for dinner.

▶ **PASTA** A low-fat carb companion for everything from greens to beans; you can simply boil it until it's soft but chewy and add olive oil and parsley. Dinner done.

83 **How long can I eat my leftover food?**

A simple rule: don't eat anything that makes you say "Whoa!" when you open the container, but don't let bad smells or fuzzy mold be your only guide. Enjoy the contents of a doggy bag you brought home or the

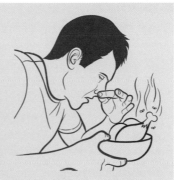

leftover Chinese within four or five days, but only if it was stowed in the fridge right away and if you make sure to get it hot all the way through. Cook groceries within three or four days, as raw meat and vegetables fall quickly under the sway of some nasty microbes. Even packaged food should be eaten within a week after you open it.

The exceptions are foods that were invented with protection against mold and bacteria in mind. Hard cheese like Cheddar or Swiss is too dense for molds to penetrate: a little surface mold can be carved off (along with about an inch of buffer); the remainder is edible. The same goes for cured meat like salami: scrub off surface mold and eat the rest. Even these, however, should sit no longer than a few weeks.

▶ **PEANUT BUTTER** A protein blast that contains the "good" kind of fat, it goes on anything—a bagel for breakfast, on a banana for a snack, with jelly and bread for lunch.

▶ **TUNA** A double-wide can will sit in the cabinet for months, ready for that night you find yourself hungry and lazy. Drain and mix in mayo, chopped celery, olives, apples, or carrots—or eat it straight out of the can.

1
2
3
4
5
6

GUYS' LIST ■

Ten rock albums every guy should own

▶ *LED ZEPPELIN II*
Led Zeppelin (1969)

▶ *SGT. PEPPER'S LONELY HEARTS CLUB BAND*
the Beatles (1967)

▶ *MUSIC FROM BIG PINK*
The Band (1968)

▶ *HOT ROCKS*
the Rolling Stones (1971)

▶ *THE DARK SIDE OF THE MOON*
Pink Floyd (1973)

▶ *THIS YEAR'S MODEL*
Elvis Costello (1978)

▶ *APPETITE FOR DESTRUCTION*
Guns N' Roses (1987)

▶ *ACHTUNG BABY*
U2 (1991)

▶ *OK COMPUTER*
Radiohead (1997)

▶ *YANKEE HOTEL FOXTROT*
Wilco (2001)

84 Five ways a home should differ from a frat house

Some guys continue to live the frat-guy lifestyle long after college, but at some point you'll want to put away the beer-pong table. Here are five elements that make a house or apartment a place fit for a grown-up:

▶ **PHOTOGRAPHS** A collection of photographs of family and friends in a prominent place gives dates and other guests something to talk about, and makes you feel connected and comfortable.

▶ **FRAMED ARTWORK** Prints and posters are fine as long as they are framed. Professional framing isn't cheap, but you can pick up extremely simple do-it-yourself frames at a big-box home store.

▶ **PERSONAL MEMORABILIA** Items you picked up at a rock concert or sporting event don't count; your childhood guitar or an oar signed by your entire crew team does, especially when displayed in a rack or hung elegantly on the wall. Artifacts or artwork you brought back from an international trip tell a story, or a framed stamp collection reveals something about you—and adds color to a room.

▶ **SERVING DISHES** If everyone who enters is happy to eat out of a bag or box, you need new friends. You don't need anything fancy: ask your parents for a tray, platter, and serving bowl they don't use anymore, or spring for something at a yard sale.

▶ **GOOD LIGHTING** You'll feel more at home if you use natural light as much as possible, maximizing your daylight with mirrors placed near windows. At night, combine tabletop lamps next to chairs and sofas for specific tasks like reading, with floor lamps placed in corners to illuminate the entire room.

85 **What should I hang on my walls?**

You don't need to haunt art galleries to dress up your walls. Art comes from any number of sources, including you: spend a day taking photographs of statues, classic buildings, barns, or close-ups

1
2
3
4
5
6

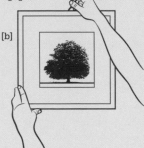

DIY 86 **How do I hang a painting or a mirror?**

1

If the piece has no hanging wire, affix one to the back with two screw eyes [a].

2

Place the piece against the wall so that your eyes meet the painting or mirror three-quarters of the way up its height. Make a light pencil mark at the center of the top of the frame [b].

3

Find the horizontal center of the frame, and let the painting hang by its wire on your finger. Make a hash mark where your finger touches the back of the piece. Measure the distance between the hash mark and the top of the frame [c].

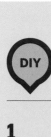

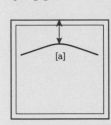

of architectural details in your area. A photography printing store can blow them up and frame them inexpensively. Do the same with evocative old family snapshots, pages from an illustrated book, or vintage vinyl record covers.

Prints made from vintage travel posters and other retro advertisements are full of color and sophistication; reprints are easily found

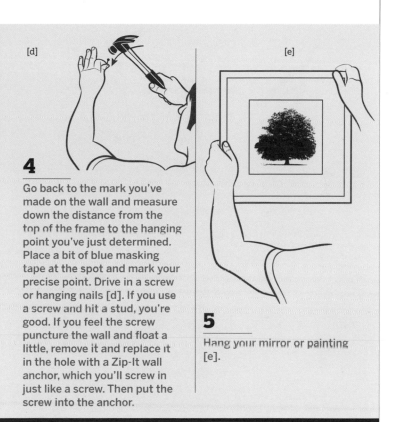

4

Go back to the mark you've made on the wall and measure down the distance from the top of the frame to the hanging point you've just determined. Place a bit of blue masking tape at the spot and mark your precise point. Drive in a screw or hanging nails [d]. If you use a screw and hit a stud, you're good. If you feel the screw puncture the wall and float a little, remove it and replace it in the hole with a Zip-It wall anchor, which you'll screw in just like a screw. Then put the screw into the anchor.

5

Hang your mirror or painting [e].

on the Internet. If you are interested in better-quality artwork, many galleries and antiques stores have original oil paintings for smaller budgets. Keep your eye out for art fairs or search the Internet for "art under $500" or for galleries that are promoting new artists with smaller works. Be guided by images you identify with.

Before you hang a picture, consider whether the artwork has a

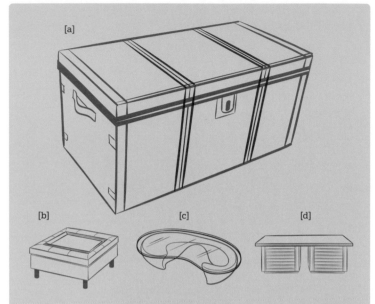

[a]

[b]   [c]   [d]

EXPERT WITNESS

87 WHAT BASIC FURNITURE SHOULD I HAVE IN MY PLACE?

DIANE OPELT
interior designer, Boston, Massachusetts

"Start with these five items: a bed, a dresser, a sleeper sofa, a comfortable chair, and a cocktail table sturdy enough to put your feet on. Don't worry about style: your coffee table can be a trunk [a], a storage unit, an ottoman with a tray [b], a large piece of sculpture that can support a glass top [c], even lobster or fruit crates you pull together to form a larger surface [d].

"One other thing: you need a place to eat other than the sofa. You should have two place settings—two dishes, matching knives, forks, salad forks, soup spoons, and teaspoons—and two quality wineglasses. That, and a box of candles, and you're all set."

horizontal or vertical shape, and whether it has counterparts in the colors already in the room. Match the art to the space: put big pieces in big areas, like an expanse of wall over a sofa, and smaller pieces in hallways and short walls.

88 **How do I shop at a yard sale?**

Be opportunistic but not impulsive. Yard sales are mostly places to snag small items: kitchen gear and other stuff that's not high on your list of desires: colanders, garlic presses, and graters. Plug anything electronic into the owner's outlet before you walk away with it.

Larger items like chairs and coffee tables can be a good buy as long as they require no repair, other than an easy coat of paint. On any item over five dollars, offer 60 percent of the asking price as a starting bid, and haggle without denigrating the item: the owner is usually happy to let his beloved possessions go cheap to someone who truly appreciates them.

89 **How do I furnish my place without spending my whole paycheck?**

Big-box home outlets are the default, but their furniture, while cheap and stylish, tends to fall apart quickly. The best deals for quality furniture are for discontinued or odd-lot items from old-school furniture retailers and department stores. Try flea markets and vintage shops, too, for well-made furniture that requires a little TLC.

GUYS' LIST

Ten items you should have in your medicine cabinet

1 | ITCH RELIEVER Keep cream on hand to smear on poison ivy and bug bites, plus a pill for bee stings or mysterious rashes.

2 | NAIL CLIPPER For basic care of fingers and toes—if you don't care what they look like, be aware that most women do.

3 | SMALL SCISSORS Handy for trimming eyebrows and nose hairs, or cutting off a week-old Band-Aid.

4 | MUSCLE BALM The two-pronged approach to a rough day on the b-ball court: an icy-hot ointment and a couple of ibuprofen, which you should also stock in bulk.

5 | FACE MOISTURIZER Unscented, with an SPF of 15. Next to clean hair and fresh breath, a smooth, supple face is the key to feeling good. (Add lip balm in winter months.)

6 | TRIPLE ANTIBIOTIC CREAM Scrapes and cuts will heal faster if you dab some on before you wrap with a Band-Aid.

7 | BAND-AIDS Get a variety of sizes, including the knee squares, which you can cut to fit smaller nicks.

8 | INDIGESTION RELIEVER Hangovers, street food, and TV football parties. Need more be said?

9 | COLD MEDICINE Bed rest and juice are great, but a combo of decongestant, painkiller, and an antihistamine will have you feelin' groovy.

10 | THERMOMETER So you know when to skip work. Simple electronic versions work faster than mercury and glass.

90 **Which houseplants will survive a brown thumb?**

There are many species out there that can survive the most punishing neglect. The snake plant (*Sansevieria trifasciata*) requires water only once or twice over the winter, more often in summer. If you want a plant that takes abuse and still blooms, try a flamingo flower (*Anthurium Pacora*), which likes low light and needs infrequent watering.

91 **Where should I position my flat-screen TV?**

Hang it at eye level since the pixels in the center of the screen are designed to be viewed straight on for the best image.

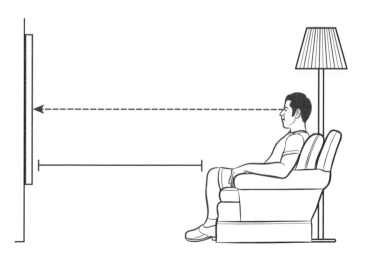

1

3
4
5
6

Ten classic movies every guy should see

1 **CASABLANCA** Humphrey Bogart at his rueful, quick-thinking best. If nothing else, you'll learn what you're supposed to look like in a white dinner jacket.
KNOW TO QUOTE: "Here's looking at you, kid"; "I am shocked, shocked to find gambling in this establishment"; "We'll always have Paris."

2 **THE GODFATHER, PARTS I AND II** The mob as a bloody, operatic family drama by Francis Ford Coppola, starring Brando and Pacino.
KNOW TO QUOTE: "I'll make him an offer he can't refuse."

3 **ONE FLEW OVER THE CUCKOO'S NEST** An insane asylum stands for America, where, as a vintage Jack Nicholson finds out, rebellion is no longer welcome.
KNOW TO QUOTE: "That's right, Mr. Martini, there's an Easter Bunny."

4 **MONTY PYTHON AND THE HOLY GRAIL** See it? You should know at least one scene verbatim.
KNOW TO QUOTE: "I'm not dead yet!"; "She turned me into a newt . . . I got better."

5 **ROCKY** A chump boxer decides he's got nowhere to go but up. So did the movie's writer and director, Sylvester Stallone.
KNOW TO QUOTE: "Adriaaaaan!"

92 **Can a TV screen be too big?**

Figure it this way: you should sit at least one and a half times as far from a screen as the length it measures from corner to corner. A forty-two-inch screen demands that the back of your sofa be at least 5.3 feet

6 | **NATIONAL LAMPOON'S ANIMAL HOUSE** It launched half a dozen comedy careers and made college fun again.
KNOW TO QUOTE: "My advice to you is to start drinking heavily"; "Toga! Toga!"; "Food fight!!"

7 | **APOCALYPSE NOW** Another Coppola masterpiece, about moral and military chaos during the Vietnam War.
KNOW TO QUOTE: "Charlie don't surf"; "Stay in the boat! Stay in the boat!"; "He said, 'If you take my picture again I'm going to kill you. And he *meant* it.'"

8 | **BLADE RUNNER** Ridley Scott reinvented both film noir and our vision of the future while Harrison Ford chased down renegade robots.
KNOW TO QUOTE: "Wake up! Time to die!"; "I've seen things you people wouldn't believe. Attack ships on fire off the shoulder of Orion. I've watched C-beams glitter in the dark near the Tannhauser Gate. All those moments will be lost in time, like tears in the rain."

9 | **THE MATRIX** Keanu Reeves discovers that reality is a computer-generated sham.
KNOW TO QUOTE: "Human beings are a disease, a cancer of this planet. You're a plague, and we are the cure."

10 | **FIGHT CLUB** A dystopic male dreamscape, with Edward Norton as a modern guy battling Brad Pitt for ownership of his soul.
KNOW TO QUOTE: "We've all been raised on television to believe that one day we'd all be millionaires, and movie gods, and rock stars. But we won't. And we're slowly learning that fact. And we're very, very pissed off."

away. A thirty-four-inch screen needs 4.3 feet. Measure the distance from wall to sofa and go shopping.

These are minimum distances at which your eye begins to make sense of the pixels; your nervous system operates on its own scale. At the store, approximate the distance between your sofa and the wall

EXPERT WITNESS

93 HOW OFTEN DO I NEED TO REPLACE MY PERSONAL ELECTRONICS?

BRIAN LAM
editor in chief of the blog Gizmodo

"You can get lost in what the latest thing is. You don't need a new thing every year, it's bad for your checkbook and for the environment. So, cool your impulses and save for a house instead. The truth is, you use your gadgets most of the time just to check e-mail. As long as the video isn't stuttering, it will play the same. When you can't stand it any longer—about every two or three years—it's time to go buy something new.

"Even then, buy last year's model. Look for sales on the Friday after Thanksgiving and after Christmas. Stay away from the cutting edge."

and ask yourself: Does a battle sequence make you queasy? Is it necessary to see LeBron James's face that big?

Lastly, consider the relative size of your furniture. A hulking television that dwarfs the unit it sits on—or the dimensions of the room itself—is not only ugly, it disorients the eye and makes viewing uncomfortable. To sum up: your screen is too big if you get more pleasure out of saying how big it is than you get actually watching it.

94 Should I get the extra warranty?

For the most part, no. Only on your laptop, and only through the company that made it, not the retailer. One year won't do either: go for three. Bigger items, like televisions and stereos, rarely break, and if they do, you don't lose important data.

95 **Where do I find cool new music?**

Internet radio has revolutionized music by allowing you to carve out your very personal niche—nichier than the radio stations that cater to, say, indie folk or blues or jazz. You tell these sites (such as Pandora, to name one) which bands you like and edit your playlist and then they recommend sounds you may not be familiar with. The Internet also gives you access to broadcast radio stations that offer new sounds without your input. (RadioTower.com indexes radio stations across the country according to genre.) You can also read music blogs that compete to post the latest updates on hot bands' recordings.

96 **How do I preserve my cell phone charge?**

The cooler the battery, the slower its charge runs out. While on the move, take the phone out of your pants pocket and away from your body heat in favor of a jacket pocket or a briefcase. If you can find a refrigerator or an operating air conditioner, give it a few minutes of concerted cooling.

If you're stranded without your charger, buy one as a last resort. Ask your hotel desk clerk if they have a compatible one, or go to a phone store that sells your phone and explain your predicament. They may let you charge up, or may even give you a charger another customer returned.

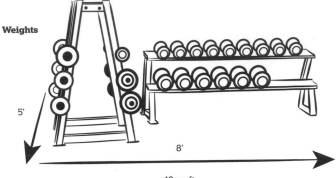

Weights

5'

8'

40 sq. ft.

97 **How do I set up a home gym?**

You build your muscles over time; a home gym should come together the same way. Mark out your gym area—it should take up no more than 10 percent of your total space—by putting down carpet or soft vinyl to protect your floor (and maybe the downstairs neighbor's quietude) and to create a separate visual and mental zone. Locate it near a closet or behind a big piece of furniture so that you have a place to roll your weights out of sight when company comes.

Start with two dumbbells and a hundred pounds of weights. Before you invest in a bench, get a Swiss ball, which requires less space, and draws more muscles into each exercise. As your muscles demand

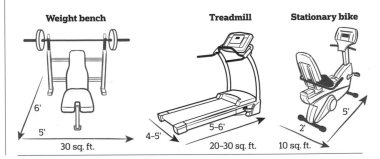

Weight bench   **Treadmill**   **Stationary bike**

6'
5'
30 sq. ft.

4–5'   5–6'
20–30 sq. ft.

5'
2'
10 sq. ft.

Five basic cleaning products you need

Grab one of each of these five items, and you'll be able to keep your place ready for visitors.

1 MULTIPURPOSE CLEANER A spray bottle of this stuff keeps grime and germs off kitchen countertops, the stove, bathroom tile, windows, even polyurethaned wood floors.

2 DISINFECTANT WIPES An industrial-strength moist towelette, these chemically treated synthetic cloths kill bacteria on surfaces from the bathroom to the kitchen.

3 PREPACKAGED DUSTING CLOTHS These creepily indestructible squares of techno-fiber capture dust without a spray, replacing the useless feather duster with something more like a tool.

4 TOILET CLEANER Toilet-cleaning technology has advanced to the point where you don't have to scrub, just let the stuff foam for a bit and flush. (In a pinch, pour in Coke, vinegar, or baking soda; let sit and scrub.) Self-cleaning systems you put on the rim of the bowl or in the tank are good if you think you'll actually replace them when needed.

5 SPOT CLEANER If you've invested in a rug, sofa, or chair, have on hand one of these intense shampoos that will stop a spill from staining the fibers or upholstery.

bigger challenges (and perhaps as you move into larger quarters), add an adjustable bench with an extension for leg curls, a barbell, and more weights. The biggest space hogs tend to be stair climbers and treadmills; if you want aerobic conditioning, get a stationary bike—or a real one, and hit the street.

GUYS' LIST

Ten classic TV series every guy should know

1 | **SPORTS NIGHT** This half-hour comedy that played like a drama ran only forty-five episodes from 1998 to 2000, but with a cast that included *Six Feet Under*'s Peter Krause and Felicity Huffman from *Desperate Housewives,* it could pull off amazing moments, many of them attempts to understand the male animal.

2 | **NYPD BLUE** This cop drama broke new ground for realism and glimpses of nudity when it debuted in 1993. But the reason to watch is Dennis Franz's hardbitten homicide detective Andy Sipowicz, whose idea of sympathy was to tell a victim's shocked colleague: "Yeah, it's a big world."

3 | **THE ODD COUPLE** Poker night, metrosexuality, three-ways with sisters—pretty much every concern of the modern man was presaged in this long-running adaptation of the Neil Simon play, starring Tony Randall as the fussbudget Felix Unger and Jack Klugman as Oscar Madison.

4 | **THE WIRE** Written by a former police reporter and a homicide detective, this cable drama is completely faithful to the reality of cops fighting drug gangs in Baltimore. But it's also a gritty microcosm of men caught up in a dog-eat-dog world.

5 | **THE PRISONER** This British series from the 1960s starred the dashing Patrick McGoohan and thematically fit in somewhere between James Bond and Franz Kafka. The nameless Number Six's attempts to escape the creepily idyllic seaside compound called "the Village" makes this the granddaddy of every show where the characters are bedeviled by unseen powers.

6 | ***BATTLESTAR GALACTICA*** In a distant futuristic civilization, robots have almost succeeded in replacing humankind—the perfect setting through which to explore present-day American society.

7 | ***MYSTERY SCIENCE THEATER 3000*** The concept is no more complicated than what your crew does when there are no good sporting events on: comedians watch bad movies and lob wisecracks at the screen. The difference is these guys turn up more mind-numbingly bad flicks than would ever show on regular TV. And their gags are funnier.

8 | ***THE TONIGHT SHOW STARRING JOHNNY CARSON*** Carson lived for good comedians, good-looking women, and those moments when his carefully planned show turned unpredictable. Rent some seasons from the early to mid seventies to get a whiff of a time in America when late-night entertainment—and the country itself—was complicated and fun.

9 | ***SATURDAY NIGHT LIVE*** The comedy of the Belushi, Aykroyd, Bill Murray, and Eddie Murphy years, in retrospect, doesn't necessarily transcend its time, and occasionally makes little sense. But that was the genius of a show that once took enormous risks and didn't seem to care if you got it.

10 | ***THE SOPRANOS*** HBO aired grown-up, smutty-mouthed dramas before Tony Soprano made his entrance, but none were so compelling, world-weary, and plain funny as the show about the Mob boss who is slowly losing his fighting spirit, and maybe his mind.

98 **How do I clean my room?**

Start by gathering all the things that don't belong in that room and putting them in piles by the door: one for the kitchen, one for the linen closet or toolbox, etc. Don't leave the room to deliver an item, or you'll get distracted. Once you have your piles working, you can allow yourself to get called away; your room will be tidier already, and you can finish up the following day with these piles as a place to start.

Once you've got your place cleaned up, keep it tidy by putting a trash can in every room. Toss everything that can go out immediately. Don't let messes pile up until the weekend: take five minutes to pick stuff up off the floor every morning. Throw dirty laundry in the hamper, hang yesterday's outfit up in the closet, and rescue shoes on the verge of going under the bed. If you bring someone home after a night out, at least your clear floor will give the impression that the entire room is clean.

99 **What do I do about roaches?**

Ridding yourself of these pests can be a fun exercise, like conducting a military campaign. First deprive the little suckers of food. Degrease the stove. Knock the crumbs out of the toaster and spirit them into the trash. Vacuum the floors and wipe up food spots. Scrub the cabinet floor where you throw away food garbage. Stay in the habit of wiping up food spills, even tiny ones, as soon as they happen.

Next, lay down a perimeter. Sprinkle boric-acid powder (or Borax cleanser) along the baseboards throughout the house. Remove your electric socket plates and blow it into the walls. (An empty ketchup squeeze bottle works well for this purpose.) Need a bigger

weapon? A substance called cypermethrin, available
online, will push back against roaches for a couple of
months. (Follow the instructions on the bottle carefully.)

During this lull, caulk up cracks—along the kitchen
baseboard and along the back of the counters. Stuff plastic shopping
bags into holes inside your cabinets, especially under the sink. If you
live in a house, rake leaves and wood away from the foundation.

Before they come back—and they will—scatter a few Roach Motel-
style traps. Then wait, and don't let them gain on you before starting
the process over.

100 **What about mice?**

For your conscience's sake, it's worth trying a
humane trap, baiting it with peanut butter and,
once you've caught something, releasing it at least a quarter mile from
your home. For your pains, you'll soon have a colony of mice in your
house. You'll never keep ahead of them with catch-and-release, or even
glue traps or snap traps. Rodent poisons have their downside—dead
mice that give up the ghost behind the fridge can smell for a day or two,
and your girlfriend may have to get over a late-night encounter with a
dying mouse, but the poisons are the only method sure to work.

101 **How do I find a compatible roommate?**

No matter how many roommates you had in college, it's different once
you get out; you'll want to choose more wisely. Your frat buddies who
like to party all night aren't going to be the best roommates when

you have to get up the next morning to go to work. You may not have cared how clean your dorm room was, but you may want your house or apartment to stay neat.

The best thing you can do is to be very up-front with people before you live with them—about your schedule, about your expectations, and especially about money for rent and utilities. And if you can't live with your buds, then look on Craigslist and find a random roommate. It sounds potentially scary, but ask around and you'll hear far more success stories than not. Remember, you don't have to be friends with your roommate. You just have to coexist happily.

102 How do I organize my closet?

Your closet doesn't need to be more complicated than a rod with a couple of shelves above. If yours lacks those basics, you can install two or three sets of one-inch board around the perimeter of your closet about fifteen inches apart vertically, then insert one-inch planks as shelving. Divide your clothes according to season, and relegate out-of-season items—sweaters in summer, white pants in winter—to a flat plastic storage tub that you can slide under your bed, or put in another out-of-the-way place.

Keep clothes that are in active rotation in the most accessible part of the closet rod and the shelves. Hang similar items together: shirts with shirts, with dress shirts and casual items in separate groups, lined up by color; organize pants the same way. Not only will the clothes look more organized, you'll be able to dress faster.

Stack sweaters, T-shirts, scarves (and anything else that doesn't hang) on shelves. Don't try to stuff too many sweaters into too small a space, and don't stack too tall, either, or the piles will tumble over.

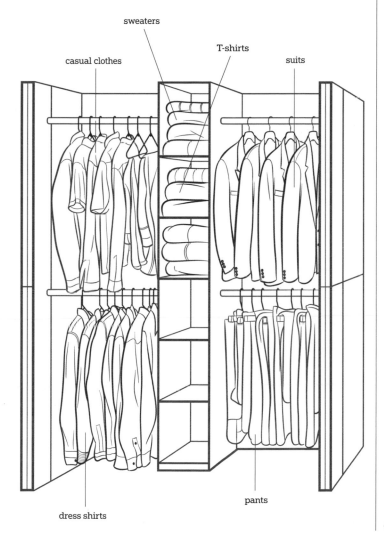

sweaters

T-shirts

casual clothes

suits

dress shirts

pants

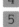

103 Which tools should I have at home?

Even if you're not handy around the house, you should have a few items to make minor fixes.

▶ **HAMMER** An eight-ounce claw hammer with a metal shaft. Skip the grooved or waffle-faced models that only mark up your surface when you miss the nail.

▶ **PLIERS** Heavy-duty electrician's pliers, with built-in wire cutters and long, rubber-insulated handles, give you more leverage and are generally more useful than the flimsy everyday pliers. Add a pair of needle-nose pliers.

▶ **SCREWDRIVERS** You'll want two sizes of Phillips head and flat head for the majority of household screws, and a set of miniature screwdrivers to replace batteries in personal electronics.

▶ **TAPE MEASURE** Buy a twenty-five-foot metal locking retractable model so you can measure objects larger than your wingspan. A three-quarter-inch tape is wide enough to stay rigid.

▶ **WRENCHES** Two adjustable wrenches with steady, comfortable adjustment screws are worth spending a tad extra on. Get a twelve-inch one for plumbing and use on other large nuts, and a smaller one for small spaces.

CAR COMPANION

104 **Which car should I buy?**

Cars are like dogs. We want them to reflect our personality, but it's more important that they fit our lifestyle. You wouldn't keep a slobbering Labrador retriever in a two-room apartment—why keep a monster pickup when you have neither a purpose for it nor parking? Decide first what you need your car for: commuting, hauling, road tripping, or running errands—all of the above? How many people are you responsible for transporting? How much car can you afford? Don't discount what your car says about you—a car should feel right—but a car that fits your needs and your wallet is man's best friend. Here's a quick summary of the kinds of cars available, with their virtues and drawbacks.

GET YOUR DRIVE ON

TYPE OF CAR	PROS	CONS	BEST FOR
Subcompact	Easy on gas, easy to park. So cheap you can afford hot options. Put a premium on imaginative designs and colors.	Safety concerns, wimpy engine, no hauling capability.	Short commutes, errands.
Compact	Extremely practical mix of space and efficiency, mileage power, versatility, lots of models to choose from, affordable.	No matter how stylish, their sheer popularity makes you blend in.	Not a hauler, but otherwise an all-around utility player.

TYPE OF CAR	PROS	CONS	BEST FOR
Midsize 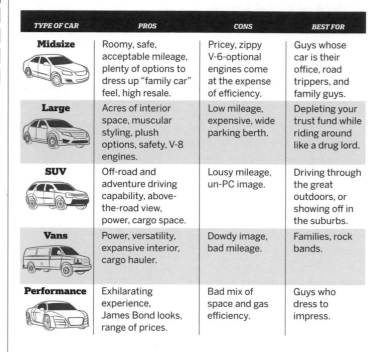	Roomy, safe, acceptable mileage, plenty of options to dress up "family car" feel, high resale.	Pricey, zippy V-6-optional engines come at the expense of efficiency.	Guys whose car is their office, road trippers, and family guys.
Large	Acres of interior space, muscular styling, plush options, safety, V-8 engines.	Low mileage, expensive, wide parking berth.	Depleting your trust fund while riding around like a drug lord.
SUV	Off-road and adventure driving capability, above-the-road view, power, cargo space.	Lousy mileage, un-PC image.	Driving through the great outdoors, or showing off in the suburbs.
Vans	Power, versatility, expansive interior, cargo hauler.	Dowdy image, bad mileage.	Families, rock bands.
Performance	Exhilarating experience, James Bond looks, range of prices.	Bad mix of space and gas efficiency.	Guys who dress to impress.

105 Manual or automatic transmission?

Any practical discussion of manuals vs. automatics usually revolves around the manual's lower cost. If guyness is the question, it's manual hands-down—they punctuate your driving with decisive thrusts and give you a place to rest your hand, evoking a magistrate on a law book. Men, besides, like to drive when they drive, and manuals give them maximum control over the car's workings. But yes, a manual transmission usually knocks a few hundred bucks off the price of a car and uses less gas. Plus, a stick shift comes in handy when you're attempting to rock the car out of snow or mud.

106 **New or used?**

The moment you drive a car off the lot, it loses thousands of dollars in value, whereas a car two years old or less has undergone the bulk of its depreciation, with plenty of wear (not to mention a year or so of warranty time) left in it. The downside of a used car is that with the industry's ever-evolving technology, you won't have the very latest in efficiency and safety equipment. Balance a used car's lower price against a new one's gas mileage or how many airbags you can afford.

107 **How do I buy a used car?**

The most important fact to know about a car you're buying is what it's worth, on the market, but also to you. Web sites and consumer magazines can give you a rough idea of its dollar value; you should have a figure in mind that represents your best offer and be prepared to walk away if it's not met. Check the car out thoroughly, take it to a mechanic, and deduct from your top price any repairs you'll have to make. Quiz the mechanic about the cost of various repairs and parts.

You're more likely to get the price you want if you pay cash, and you should expect at any rate to pay with a cashier's check, certified by your bank. If a private seller is "asking" for a certain price or listed the car as "OBO," begin the negotiation by offering 10 to 20 percent less; stay closer to a price advertised as "firm." It's okay to cite particular problems that will take money to fix, but don't disparage the car in general.

Once you've made a deal, get the signed title as well as a bill of sale outlining the terms of the deal with both parties' names and addresses and the price. Check with your local motor-vehicle bureau about who gets the license plates.

108 How do I know I'm not buying a clunker?

Before you go see the car, search the Web to read up on any specific problems the model you're buying is prone to—weak brakes, cheap interior materials—and inspect them carefully before you buy. Ask the seller if the car has been in an accident. (You can ask for the car's accident history to be run on an Internet service.)

When you go to see the car, look for undue wear and evidence that the car has been in a crack-up (which can introduce other problems, such as a bent frame). Push the car down at each corner and watch to make sure the bouncing stops quickly after you've let go. The steering wheel should have an inch of play, no more, when the car is parked.

When you drive the car, listen for rumbling or squealing as you turn. The automatic transmission should shift the car immediately into gear, without a lag or thump. Examine the exterior for lumpy or nonmetallic portions, which might indicate bodywork resulting from an accident, and for rust. Press on the footwell floors to detect holes or soft spots. Check the tires for bald spots or uneven wear.

What's okay? A battery that looks like it's seen better days won't cost much to replace. A little squeaking in the brakes is normal. Some squealing when you turn on the ignition is a loose fanbelt.

109 **What's the best way to work with a car dealer?**

Cars are one of those commodities, like houses and airplane seats, that have no firm, objective value. The price is determined by how hard you shop. Make a list of all the dealers within a manageable distance. Favor big dealerships, which make their money by selling in volume. Call first, let them know you are comparing prices at different dealerships, and get their best offer. Record the name of the person you spoke to. Now pick the two or three dealerships. Have a good meal, be rested, and head for the dealership. If possible, bring a friend.

Be aware that every phase of buying a car is part of the negotiation: from questions about how you're going to finance the purchase to seemingly casual discussions about your old car. The corollary is that everyone you talk to, whether they are called a closer, a manager, or a trade-in appraiser, is a salesperson. Don't give them any information that's not about the price you want to spend for the car you're looking at.

Your ultimate power is to walk out at any moment. Decline invitations to sit down until you have a deal. When you do sit down, have in front of you the price that got you to stay. Many figures will be thrown at you; don't depart from the one that you agreed to.

110 **How do I change my oil?**

You can take your car in and get your oil changed, or you can easily do it yourself by following these steps:

1

Find a flat spot in your garage or on your driveway. Jack up your car—or else put it on some old cinder blocks—and keep your cell handy to dial 911 in case you're under the car when it falls on you.

2

Slide under the car and locate the oil drain plug. Place a pan under the plug to catch the old oil. With the car off and cool, loosen the plug with a socket wrench and let the oil drain. Stay nearby to reposition the pan as the rush of oil slows.

3

Replace the oil plug gasket [a], giving it a film of oil to help it seal [b]. Tighten it, first with your fingers to make sure the

threads are staying on line, then with the socket wrench.

4

Find the oil filter. Put the pan under the filter and unscrew it with your filter wrench. Make sure the old gasket hasn't clung to the filter mount. Screw the new filter in by hand [c].

5

Now open the hood of the car. Loosen the oil filler cap and add new oil [d]. Your user's manual will tell you how much the engine takes. After refilling, run the engine for a bit, turn it off, and check the oil level [e].

6

Bring the waste oil to a recycling center or drop it off with your mechanic.

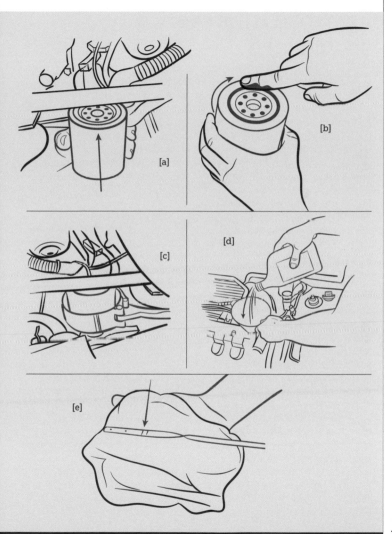

[a]

[b]

[c]

[d]

[e]

GUYS' LIST

Five road trips every guy should take

1 VERMONT ROUTE 100 Start out from the classic ski village of Stowe on Route 100 in mid to late September when the leaves are blazing, reflected in a distractingly picturesque river you follow for much of the way. These hundred miles through the Green Mountain National Forest and up to the cliff-walled pass at Smugglers' Notch aren't the longest road trip, but let the locals pass you and make it last as long as you can.

2 CALIFORNIA ROUTE 1 A cliché that nonetheless applies, this 125-mile stretch along the coast is the Pebble Beach of drives. The highlight is Big Sur, where the mountains crash into the Pacific; for much of it, you and your passengers will be stunned into silence.

3 PIERRE, SOUTH DAKOTA, TO MOUNT RUSHMORE The trip from the state capital—you'll never forget that one again—south on U.S. Route 83 and then west using I-93 as your directional (but not your only road) takes you across

two grassland preserves and the moonscape of Badlands National Park to Rapid City, and Teddy, Tom, Abe, and George looking out at you from the Black Hills. If this two-hundred-mile trek isn't out there enough, you can continue into the Black Hills National Forest.

4 U.S. ROUTE 6 Portions of this two-laner that run from the California border through Nevada, Utah, crossing the Continental Divide at Loveland Pass, and ending in Denver may be the most haunting desert and mountain scenery that you can see by car. There's nothing wrong with you that this 1,500-mile trek won't cure.

5 THE ALASKAN HIGHWAY In Dawson Creek, British Columbia, the once rugged, now completely manageable, but still remote Alaskan Highway starts its northwesterly journey through Yukon Territory and into the Alaskan heartland. Append the extra jaunt from Seattle through B.C. and on to Fairbanks for a tidy 2,300 miles.

111 **What kind of options should I pay for?**

The safety options are not only sensible, they're also cost-effective, since a car with the full safety package retains its value better and may cost less to insure. The same goes for air-conditioning: you might be able to live without it, but you'll eat the cost when you sell the car or trade it in. The more economical the car you buy, the more options you'll be able to afford: the more luxurious the base car, the faster the options pile on the price.

112 **What makes a good mechanic?**

Ask for recommendations from friends and family members who are happy with their mechanic. You're looking for one that's not only good but honest, too. When you visit, look for an orderly, if not exactly spotless, work bay. The office where you pay your bill may be a pigsty as long as the place where your car is going to be repaired looks like the arena of a professional. You'll notice belts hung on the wall, boxes stacked neatly, and machinery rationally placed. There should be at least two mechanics working in the shop—any fewer, and the shop is likely overloaded and won't get to your car promptly.

When you bring in your car for service, a good mechanic will ask a few questions about the trouble you're having, or about work you want done. He won't have an issue with giving you estimates for different possible repair strategies (and he'll call with a firm estimate once he's diagnosed the problem). When you return for your car, he'll warn you about repairs you may need soon, for example, brake pads

1
2
3
4
5
6

Ten classic cars any guy would want to own

1 FORD MUSTANG The original iteration is still the closest the American motor industry got to a classic touring sportster. The Mustang inspired a new category of "pony" cars—relatively small, muscle-y models with sweet lines. So many were manufactured, you may still be able to find one in your price range.

2 PLYMOUTH BARRACUDA The 'Cuda Hemi's E-body, with a larger engine bay accommodating its 5.7-liter engine, mixes pure lines and American power. A vintage '71 is so fast, pretty, and sought after that a mint example can go for more than a Ferrari at auction.

3 CHEVY NOVA SS Something about the plain lines ending in a stubby rear end captures the seventies aesthetic perfectly, while communicating the car's single-minded attention to power.

4 DATSUN Z CAR Fast, exotic, and cheap at the time, Datsun's "poor man's Jag" was such a surprise hit that, as the commercials once boasted, used models were as expensive as new ones.

5 CHEVY EL CAMINO Bill Clinton remade the redneck reputation of these low-riding cars with an Impala front and a pickup rear when he implied that he'd nailed a lady friend in the bed of his. As car enthusiasts cry for American carmakers to restore the "elco" or its cousin, the Ford Ranchero,

or tires if yours look worn. If he trusts you to bring the car back to him instead of urgently recommending that the work be done right away, you can probably trust him.

to production, it's not too late to appreciate the original McCoy.

6 | **MGB** This growly, well-mannered sportster fell behind in performance terms in the 1960s, but was so beloved by Brits and Americans alike that it has hung on to become a classic. Drive gently, perhaps with a pair of gloves and a tweed cap.

7 | **VW BEETLE** Slow, noisy, and bare-boned, the Bug is nonetheless a snap to fix, and its ungainly hump is nothing less than iconic.

8 | **MERCEDES-BENZ 560 SL** The late-eighties SLs are riding the leading edge of classic, meaning it's just the time to catch one before they become no more affordable than the museum-priced 300SL "Gullwing" coupes.

9 | **PORSCHE 356 COUPE** So perfectly designed and manufactured, this forty-year-old "tubby" is not only perhaps the most beautifully zaftig body ever made, but is still practical for getting around town, with more than decent gas mileage and a ready, if easily tired engine.

10 | **BMW 2002** The two-door entry in BMWs "new class" of 1960s cars was reviewed by one critic as a "small crate with its few fittings, old-fashioned engineering, hard ride and curiously designed door frames." It made BMW's name outside Germany, and by the time it was retired in the mid-seventies it had become a classic.

1
2
3
4
5
6

113 **How do I check my belts?**

The wear on an engine belt is pretty obvious. You'll see fraying, cracks, or small tears in the belt long before it fails. The belt that can do the most harm to your engine if it goes, however, is buried deep in the engine. It's the timing belt and it should be replaced around the sixty-thousand-mile mark on most cars (check your manual).

3

Work

Once upon a time a guy was defined by what he did—
a cop, a bus driver, a stockbroker, an artist. You took
on the role completely because you joined when you
were young and mastered a set of skills on your way to
the gold watch. In this generation, jobs are things we
put on and take off like a pair of jeans, and what
defines a guy is how he copes with changes. ▶

1
2
3
4
5
6

GETTING THE JOB

114 **What should I do with my life?**

Ask what kind of atmosphere you want to spend the next forty or so years in. What kind of people do you admire? What provides satisfaction: Helping others? Building wealth? Creating new things? How much do you like risk? Travel? Late nights? What do you do when you can do anything—Watch TV? Go for a hike? Shop for clothes?

These questions may lead you to a specific industry—bioengineering, nonprofit, food service, or film. But remember that every industry is a microcosm of the economy at large: Movie studios need accountants and hairdressers as well as actors. Restaurants need interior designers and suppliers as well as cooks. Just because you don't play an instrument doesn't rule out a career in music as a marketer or an electrician. Whatever your interest, you likely have skills that apply. You just have to find out where those skills and your interests merge.

Next, find out what life in that career is really like. Find people in the profession you're aiming for. Read their biographies in magazines or newspapers. Write to or meet with anyone whose career you admire. Ask them how they got there, how they spend their day. (Don't ask for a job—if they have a place to offer you, they'll be flattered enough by your interest to mention it.) If you can afford to, take an internship in the field to get an inside look at its daily routines. If you're still enthusiastic, you'll already be on your way.

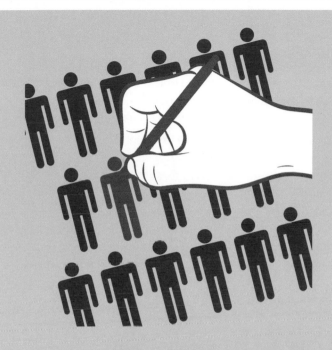

115 HOW DO I SELL MYSELF?

ALLISON HEMMING
president of The Hired Guns, a head-hunting agency

"It's important to curate and develop your personal brand. Your personal brand is the essence of you—the attributes that you want people to know about you, including the successes you've had. Most people go on too long, or are too wonky, when they explain who they are. You should be able to tell it in an authentic, simple story about yourself—think about how you'd explain yourself at a cocktail party. That way, other people can tell your story for you, and pretty soon you'll become watercooler fodder."

1
2
3
4
5
6

116 **How do I find my dream job?**

Résumés, cover letters, and thank-you notes are important, but nothing helps get you hired like a personal connection to the person who is hiring. The advent of Internet job sites has only reinforced this truism by overwhelming employers with applications from numerous job seekers of various levels of skill.

Any serious job hunter, therefore, will shamelessly exploit his connections to the company he wishes to join. Draw a chart with your name on one side and your dream employer on the other and map your progress. Then contact professors, parents, friends' parents, fellow alumni of your high school or college, golfers you once caddied for—anyone you have the *cojones* to call—and inform them of your job search. Ask if they know anyone in your target company, and if they could introduce you.

117 **What if I don't want an office job?**

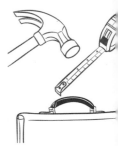

Non-office jobs often require a particular skill or talent: funeral directors, landscape architects, elevator repairmen, and pilots all submit to extensive training or apprenticeships or both. A formal degree isn't always necessary, though experience alone no longer credentials you the way it once did. Even in artistic fields, a graduate degree in creative writing, painting, or dance can make the difference between a paying job in those fields and being a starving artist. If you want to avoid the nine-to-five life, just make sure you're willing to put in the effort to get the proper skills.

118 HOW DO I START MY OWN BUSINESS?

BRIAN TWIBELL
CEO, Red Vision

"I started my first business when I was twenty-six. I had no clue what I was getting into. It succeeded because I kept at it, was passionate, and had some luck. But I also learned a few rules for the next one."

▶ **GET SOME EXPERIENCE** "I was young, but I had worked in a bank long enough to get a firm grounding and develop my ideas. Also, know what you're not and fill the void. I was the marketing and business-oriented guy. My cofounder was a phenomenal software developer."

▶ **PROVIDE SOMETHING UNIQUE** "You can make a living from a pet shop business, but if you want to build something very rewarding financially, there's no point producing something that exists. The key component is the idea itself—a service that nobody's performing, finding an underserved market or a new technology that reduces labor. Then, think the idea through: the whole customer experience, the supply chain, and who your third-party partners might be."

▶ **SURVIVE ON SWEAT EQUITY** "It's very hard for a young person with little experience to raise capital. Don't go for professional investors until you have a product and a client. In the meantime, unless you have a rich uncle, you need to bootstrap it. Do as much of the work as you can yourself, take a minimal salary, and raise funds as you grow. The longer you wait to bring in investors, the less of the company you'll have to give up."

▶ **PUT THINGS IN WRITING** "Small businesses are like rock bands. They sometimes collapse in the midst of succeeding. It's not a lack of trust but too much that breaks you up. Agreeing on the partners' responsibilities, compensation, and exit strategy forces you to discuss these issues before they threaten the business."

119 How do I write a résumé when I don't have a lot of experience?

When you first enter the workforce, your résumé, which is a formal list of the jobs you've held, is a bit of a contradiction. But the format can be adapted for the first-time job seeker.

▶ **START WITH YOUR GOAL** Begin your résumé with a single sentence outlining the type of job you are seeking. You can tailor this for each prospective employer.

▶ **EMPHASIZE ACCOMPLISHMENTS** Think creatively about experiences that shaped you or that showcased your leadership or salesmanship. Volunteer and charitable activities, travel, clubs you founded or held office in—it's all fair game if you can relate it concisely to the type of work you're pursuing. (Sports feats should be listed separately under "Interests and Hobbies," but this is where being manager of a team will work in your favor.)

▶ **AWARDS** Obviously, you want to list student government or fraternity elections you won. Include high school achievements only if they are particularly relevant or impressive. (Sorry, high scores on arcade games don't count.)

▶ **USE EMPLOYER-FRIENDLY KEYWORDS**
Explain your triumphs using words that translate to the workplace. Avoid passive language like "did," "has been," "was." Instead use active words like "responsibly," "lead," "managed," "built," and

"founded"—"Managed bell-ringing club and built membership to fifty in two years," not "Had experience in growing membership of bell-ringing club."

▶ **PLAY UP EDUCATIONAL DATA** In addition to the degree you earned and the institution that granted it, list your GPA (if it's above a 3.0), your making the dean's list, any awards, grants, fellowships, or published papers, and even your SAT scores if they will impress.

▶ **BEEF UP YOUR DESIGN** Leave plenty of white space, even at the cost of including every last astonishing detail. Your design should be traditional—look at résumé templates available online, and ask successful friends and relatives for theirs, too. Remember that you'll be sending the résumé by e-mail, in some cases pasted into the body of the message, so keep the formatting simple.

120 How do I ace a phone interview?

These days, employers often make their first cut by phone. The good news: you don't have to make sense while dummied up in a suit or worry about shaking hands with sweaty palms. The bad news: for much of the interview, you're talking into empty space, unable to read your interviewer.

Take a few measures, therefore, in order to ground yourself. Have in front of you a clock, your résumé, notes on the particular job you're interviewing for (including, lest you forget, the interviewer's name), and pen and paper. As you're asked each question, jot down the key point and focus your answer on that. Breathe, smile, and above all speak slowly—for the interviewer's sake, and to give yourself time to formulate thoughts without having to resort to "ums" or "you knows."

121 What are the elements of a good cover letter?

A cover letter should interpret your résumé, spinning the raw data listed into a short, compelling narrative about your career so far and particularly how that career relates to the job on offer—all in four or five concise sentences. Write your letter with the advertisement describing the job in front of you and pull out those experiences that directly apply. You can't be too explicit: "seeking experienced programmer" should correspond to a line in your cover letter saying "with more than five years' experience as a programmer . . ." If your background doesn't match the qualifications they're looking for, point to the skills—salesmanship, people management, financial acumen—that will translate directly to the job at hand.

122 How do I prepare for a job interview?

By the time they meet you face-to-face, your prospective employers know a lot about you: your work history plus whatever the person who recommended you told them. Close the information gap by doing a quick Internet search on your interviewer and other key players at the company. Take note of where company officers have worked, gone to school, or grew up so you can capitalize on anything you have in common. Call friends to find someone who has worked for or knows the person. If you can find someone who has worked for the company, or even a current employee whom you think you can trust, call and ask what she would want to know if she were in your spot. Find out if there are any unexpected parts to the job, or things you should know to put yourself ahead of the game for the interview. Most of all remember to go in calm and confident. Give thoughtful answers that show you've done your homework on the company, and you'll ace it. (For what to wear, see page 128.)

123 What do I say when they ask about my biggest flaw?

Disguise a strength as a weakness: Say you are too much of a perfectionist and don't take your own mistakes well. Say you make decisions swiftly, and at times you could seek more consensus. Or that you speak your mind when you see something could be done better, and don't always observe the politics of what you are saying. Don't be disingenuous, but frame your drawback by mentioning its upside.

124 How do I respond to an invitation to critique the company?

Occasionally an interviewer will invite you to offer suggestions on the company's products and what you'd do differently. You may be tempted to show off your bright ideas, but this question can lead into a minefield. A too brutally honest critique will likely offend someone—even the person sitting across the desk from you. Softballing the question could make it look as if you have nothing to contribute. Start any critique with an ample list of what you admire about the company's efforts. Then mention a few areas where you think things could be improved and where your background has prepared you to be a positive force. Don't allow yourself to be led into criticizing particular strategies. If you say that you don't know enough about what guided specific decisions, you'll only be telling the truth.

125 **How do I negotiate my pay?**

Once you get a firm offer and express your excitement at coming to work, but before you say yes, take a day to consider what you would like to make in salary and how that matches up with the offer you've just received. Do some homework online about what people

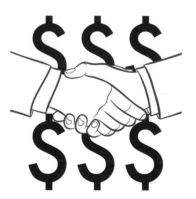

in equivalent positions with equivalent experience make. If you have been in touch with the previous occupant of the position, feel free to call and get a sense of what you should ask for.

When you call your new employer back, be upbeat and positive but ask whether the salary is negotiable. If the answer is yes, name a figure slightly above what you can settle for. Justify it by citing your experience and by what others in your position are making. Once you've stated your case, be quiet in order to

force the firm's negotiator to respond.

Salary is not always negotiable. Be prepared to accept other forms of compensation, like more vacation time, or to get the employer to agree to an evaluation after a set period of time that will reopen the question of your pay. It's a good idea to have your backup list of perks ready so you can immediately respond to the negotiator's refusal.

Now ask for the deal in writing, or at least in an e-mail, and when you get it, commit to the job as soon as you can.

126 **Do I have to take a company drug test?**

If you've celebrated your big offer with an ill-advised indulgence, your only real ally is time. Try to delay the test at least a day, if not a week—if you're currently employed, you might say your current boss asked for a day or two to make a counteroffer. If you're sure you're going to fail a test, go to Human Resources and explain that you mistakenly whooped it up at a party a couple of nights before. Offer to submit to random tests in the future. Or you can hope what you took is not what they are looking for. Companies are most concerned about defending themselves against highly addictive drugs that cause employees to steal. When one young Wall Street recruit asked a company doctor if marijuana would show up in his urine, the doctor answered, "Not as cocaine it won't."

ON THE JOB

127 **How do I tell my boss he or she is wrong?**

The boss doesn't pay you to be a mindless drone. Your views are part of what you are hired to provide, and airing them exhibits leadership. But to show you're not simply bucking authority, be ready to offer alternatives. Write them up in a memo—don't criticize at a meeting—with a note asking your boss whether a suggestion would be welcome. You'll help your case if you weave into your plan a previous move the boss has made—or better yet, a principle she has taught you.

128 **How do I compete with the corporate climbers?**

There's no use denying that suck-ups and credit hogs—guys who make promotion an end in itself—often end up in charge. Corporate life, like life anywhere else, is not always fair. Rather than fight the realities, consider what the boss sees in your rival. The guy is likely in the office regularly, if not constantly; that's why the boss thinks he knows what's going on. He's not afraid to offer his opinions—even if they are swiped from others. He dresses well—okay, it's all part of his facade, but every day he looks suited up and ready. He makes himself indispensable to the boss by providing numbers, appearing out of nowhere when a crisis hits, and moving in on projects above his pay grade—whatever it takes to make himself look good.

You wouldn't stoop to this guy's worst behavior. But be aware of what he does right. Consider what the boss thinks of you, show up every day ready to work, be positive, and be at the boss's elbow in a crisis and you'll outgun the schemer at his own game.

129 **What can I do to expand my network?**

By all means take advantage of business-oriented sites (like Plaxo or LinkedIn) as well as Facebook and other social sites. And don't simply connect with people: contact them for advice, congratulate them on promotions, and generally stay in their virtual field of vision. But don't rely on these sites; mingle the old-fashioned way. Join a professional

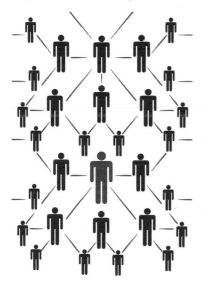

organization and volunteer at their events. Help a friend throw an industry event like a cocktail hour or corporate run. Attend parties where industry folks, especially those from other companies, are going to be. Sure, you should get people's cards and hand out a few of your own, but the point of these exercises is not to ask for a job or even talk business, but to become a face that everyone knows.

Let your network grow.

1
2
3
4
5
6

130 **How should I behave when I'm the boss?**

You've been promoted because your higher-ups have faith in you. Have the same faith in yourself and, more important, have the same faith in those below you. Hand out praise often and in public—the achievements of those who report to you reflect on your leadership. Mentor those with less experience, prepping them to take your place— you won't get promoted again until the company has confidence it can replace you. Help them to promote their careers so that grateful alums of your department begin to populate the company and your industry.

131 **How do I supervise my former colleagues?**

Don't make excuses for your new power. Most people want to be led, and are happy to have you take the heat of responsibility. If you've worked with your new reports as a peer for some time before being promoted, begin your first meeting with a short statement thanking your colleagues for their support and leave it at that.

If one of your more ambitious underlings suddenly attempts to outshine you—say, by going directly to the boss with ideas he or she hasn't cleared with you—remind him that since you know more about the company's plans, he or she should check with you before offering innovations. Then, if the ideas are good, support them. If you're constantly challenged by one former peer, take the person to lunch and explain that she is making life miserable for both of you, and her option is to get in line or leave.

132 **Can I tell my boss to stuff it?**

Yes, but take time to compose yourself so you don't explode. Think through the reasons that you feel the boss's request is unfair—you've already worked three weekends in a row or can't take on another big project without adequate help. (If you can't come up with any reasons, consider whether you are overreacting or feel stressed by something outside work.) Come up with a plan to get the work done in a rational manner. Go talk to the boss in person, prefacing your remarks by saying something like, "You know I'd do anything for the company, but ..." You may not have to say very much. When the boss is pushing you past your endurance point, he or she probably knows it already.

133 **How do I stay on my boss's good side?**

Two things a boss hates: being surprised and feeling unsupported. Never let her get news, pleasant or unpleasant, from another source if you knew it already. Not only don't you get to control the fallout, but the boss will feel betrayed.

Stay in touch and focused on the boss's problem. This extends to your physical whereabouts. In general, she should know where to find you. Leave a note on your computer screen or let a nearby colleague know where you're going when you leave your workstation for more than a few minutes.

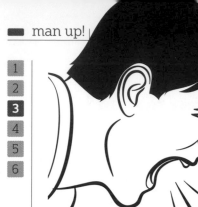

1
2
3
4
5
6

134 **How do I respond when the boss screams at me?**

Don't allow the blowup on one side to turn into a blowup on both sides. Breathe deeply (to prevent yourself from losing your temper— or laughing) and maintain eye contact without glaring. Don't speak until you are invited to respond, at which point it's better to suggest a way to fix the problem than to defend your actions. When the blowup is over, don't storm out, hide, or leave the office before quitting time (or before you've taken steps to make the boss happy), but make your-self scarce as soon as it is politic to do so. No one wants to work in a volatile environment, so you have to ask yourself if this was a onetime thing, or something that happens repeatedly. If you're being chewed out all the time for things that are not your fault, speak to another superior in the office to find a way to handle the situation.

135 **What can I do to advance my career?**

"Start looking the day you're hired" is an exaggeration, but one that contains a kernel of truth. It's the rare employee who sticks around until retirement these days, and companies return the favor by looking outside their halls when filling the plum jobs. Even a lateral move can improve your standing by confirming that you're a sought-after commodity.

That doesn't mean you should move indiscriminately. Switching jobs more than once every two to three years creates the impression that you're a professional butterfly, or bad news. If you're not getting a raise, the new place should offer more prestige or a better record of promoting from within. Employers are aware of any noncompete clauses in your current contract, or restrictions on stealing clients.

Last, don't seek out offers just to wring concessions from your current employer. Once you declare yourself a free agent, staying put in a position created to please you is nothing but awkward for both sides.

136 **How do I know when it's time to leave a job?**

If you've been at your current shop for three years without a promotion, or if a complete doofus you have no respect for gets promoted over you, it's time to leave. Alternatively, if you've been promoted repeatedly and sent on every out-of-town mission but suddenly find yourself left out of every meeting, you should take the hint. You may also need to move on if the guy who hired you stumbles. If your boss gets fed to the lions, and the new regime comes in with guns blazing to "move the organization in another direction," the writing is on the wall.

137 **How do I quit?**

Tell your immediate superior that you're leaving as soon as you know you're going to accept another offer. Do this in person, making an appointment if necessary, and bring along a written letter of resignation. (Keep a copy for your own file, annotating it with the date you began working, and your starting and finishing salary—this information is crucial the next time you update your résumé.) As you present the news, be polite but firm, putting only what the boss needs to know in the best light—that you've learned a lot, but you are moving on because your new job offers you an opportunity to raise the level of your game. And let the boss know first, lest the news spread before you can deliver it the way you want to. Remember, he gave you a chance once, and you may need his goodwill again.

Don't just be nice; be responsible. Leave a memo detailing the status of your current projects, and make yourself available by phone to answer any questions. Then make a clean break. Two weeks' notice is standard for entry-level and middle-management jobs. Whatever date is determined, stick to it. You owe the boss no more than this, and staying longer only allows more time for bad feelings to crop up.

138 **What is the best way to give constructive criticism?**

Consider first whether the person really wants your opinion at all—sometimes a colleague will ask for your read on her actions when she just wants you to help her rationalize them. Before you start problem-solving for her, ask outright: "Are you asking for my input?" Your colleague may just want to vent.

If she seems to truly want your take, make sure you build from what she did right. Identify her reasons for doing what she did and point out that following her heart or looking out for her own feelings or time is important. Then suggest ways it could have been handled better. If she bristles at the idea that she fell short, try couching your misgivings by strategizing with her on how to deal with any repercussions or criticisms she should expect.

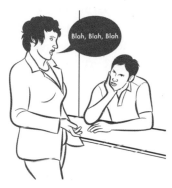

139 **How do I stop a blabbermouth at work?**

Chatting at your cubicle with a colleague can be a bonding experience or an indispensable form of brainstorming. But when a colleague shows up daily to gab for extended periods, deal with him or her promptly. "I could talk about this stuff all day," you can say, "but I've got to get back to work." If the subject of your chat is legitimate company business, suggest that you schedule a meeting to include others who are involved in the project. Your last resort, before asking a more senior person to speak to the chatterer, is to visit the person at his cubicle and explain that you feel uncomfortable with the behavior. The worst that could happen is they give you the silent treatment.

140 **How do I make a good presentation?**

Give up your written text. Come up with three words that key the essential points you want to make, and write them on index cards. On each card, add two words or phrases that will remind you of the subtopics within each point. If you need to quote a person or document word for word, write the quote on the reverse of the card that pertains to that portion of the speech. Then, armed with no more than these cards, walk your audience through your presentation.

With no text to read from, you'll be able to make eye contact, use body language, use examples creatively, reverse direction, and even stumble over your words, communicating both your depth of knowledge and your humanity. By condensing your speech to just three points, you'll also be less likely to talk beyond your audience's attention span. If you're slated to speak for longer, open the floor to Q&A. Asking for "questions on what I've covered so far" can also buy you time if your mind goes blank.

Get some physical exercise before you go on, even if you have to do push-ups in your suit backstage, in order to relax (especially your shoulders, which hike up when you're nervous). If you find yourself getting bound up, drop your shoulders, take a deep breath, and give the audience a cryptic smile.

141 **Should I date someone from work?**

The workplace is a nearly ideal venue to familiarize yourself with a member of the opposite sex—to appreciate her taste in clothes and friends, judge how she acts under pressure, steal glances at her figure, and breathe deeply of her pheromones. Plus, as Jim and Pam found out on *The Office*, you'll be sure to have plenty of workmates dying to come to the wedding.

Bonus: you never have to scheme to get close to her: you see each other practically every day. But therein lies the complication. If your romance sours, you run the risk of poisoning what was a perfectly good professional relationship (plus your chances of dating anyone else at the office). Your company may also frown on intramural dating. Make sure your feelings for the person are worth the risk of having to find a new job.

If you are still interested after a few months of pining, ask her discreetly if she'd like to do something one evening, or over the weekend. If that leads to more dates, try not to change your behavior toward one another at work: No butt-whacking or making faces at meetings. Don't start working late to conceal the fact that you're heading in the same direction each night. Absolutely refrain from hanky-panky on company premises. On the other hand, don't avoid each other: go to lunch in company with others and seek each other out for chats. If someone confronts you with suspicions, don't lie; unless it's your boss, say your private life is your business. But you may also want to start looking for another job.

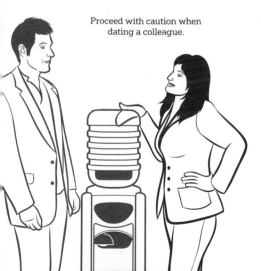

Proceed with caution when dating a colleague.

1
2
3
4
5
6

THE UNIFORM

142 What do I wear to a job interview?

If you're looking for an office job, a suit is absolutely necessary—experts disagree only on whether navy or gray is the most appropriate color. For jobs that involve manual labor or fieldwork, you can't go wrong with a shirt and tie with khakis, though you may want to dress in a way that suggests you're ready to work that day if necessary—say, a polo shirt tucked in over a white T-shirt, worn with jeans or work pants with a belt. No matter how sloppy the job, your interview outfit should represent your work: clean and well organized.

143 How many suits do I need?

You should own one suit for every day of the week your job requires you to wear one, plus one. If the job demands a suit every workday, your minimum is six: the extra will be in the cleaners, or out of season. If you wear a suit just once a week, that's two suits to you; if you're never required to wear a suit, you need just one, for special occasions. Replace your suit at least every two years, and keep it clean and pressed in a hang bag in the closet.

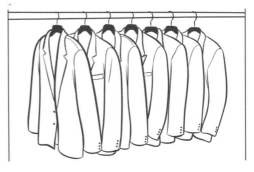

144 How do I wear a pocket handkerchief?

A neat line of white handkerchief showing a spare quarter inch is all this effect requires. A big poof of silk exploding from your jacket's breast pocket will make you look like you're posing—as what is not even clear.

For a single-point pocket square, lay a simple, fifteen-inch white cotton or silk square down in front of you, points up and down so that it presents itself like a diamond [a]. Fold the bottom point up to meet the top point [b]. Now you have a triangle. Turn the left-hand corner to the right so that the point lands halfway along the bottom side of the triangle [c]. Repeat with the right-hand corner [d]. Tuck the pocket square into the breast pocket of your suit or sport coat.

For a double-point pocket square, start the same as a single point, but offset the two points in your initial fold so that both top and bottom points are distinct. Then proceed to fold and tuck as above.

Once you've slipped it into your pocket, hands off. If you can't leave it alone, leave it at home.

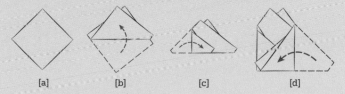

[a]   [b]   [c]   [d]

145 If I have just one suit, what should it be?

A dark gray suit in a year-round weight is the men's version of the little black dress—it goes to weddings, job interviews and, without a tie, out on the town. Stick with a classic cut from a major label.

146 **Can I afford a custom suit?**

A custom, or bespoke, suit was once something you worked your way up to, like the corner office. Nowadays, there is the Hong Kong tailor. For about the cost of a designer suit, these itinerant tailors measure you up and send you a custom-made suit in the mail. Hong Kong tailors, so called because their workshops are in Asia, announce their arrival in a major city by word of mouth by putting out flyers with the ragtag look of ransom notes. When they hit town, they set up shop in a hotel room, take measurements and orders, and send the specs back east to be turned into suits. The results show up in your mail box about two months later.

What you don't get for that price is Old World service. When visiting a Hong Kong tailor, be prepared to snap off answers about your choice of fabric, cut, number of buttons. Wear and bring along pictures of suits you admire or look good in.

147 **What do I wear for an office job?**

Before you invest in a wardrobe, it pays to reconnoiter. Even big-city law firms don't demand a suit every day. In some industries, suits are all but taboo, or are reserved for the employees who woo clients, while "creative" shows up in vintage T-shirts and distressed jeans. It can vary within an industry, too: some Internet firms have a "surf's up!" shorts-and-tee vibe, while others harbor ranks of programmers in identical French blue shirts and dark gray pants.

These workplace "uniforms" make shopping for clothes and dressing in the morning mighty convenient. But don't feel constrained to dress like everyone else. If suits are your thing, don one at your pleasure. If you can't think except in jeans, wear them, and keep a good suit on a hanger in case your top client comes by for lunch. If you find yourself constantly at odds with the dress code, you may want to rethink your line of work or your place of employ.

148 Are short sleeves acceptable with a suit?

Once reserved for NASA denizens, short-sleeved shirts have surfed to fashionability again on the backs of hipsters who treasure a sort of mid-twentieth-century dorkiness. For wear under a suit, however, short-sleevers are not advisable. For one thing, they rob your look of the stylish quarter inch of sleeve peeking from your jacket cuff. Inevitably, too, you'll want to take your jacket off at work without looking like Dilbert.

149 How do I pick a suit fabric?

▶ **COTTON** Comfortable against the skin no matter how sweltering the weather, cotton suits are the right choice for summer workdays and occasions, like outdoor hot-weather weddings, when you want to be informally formal. Higher-end haberdashers have focused on the khaki suit in recent years, creating sharply tailored versions of the traditionally dowdy-cut khaki suit, increasing your options, and extending the opportunities to wear cotton for clubbing (with an open-necked shirt).

▶ **WOOL** Wool is wrinkle-, stain-, and water-resistant, it's warm yet light, supple, and plentiful. Were they not the most oblivious creatures on earth, you might suspect that sheep grow their coats with our suits in mind.

▶ **FLANNEL** A winter-weight fabric that makes for a softer feel but a bit of a stiffer look.

▶ **GABARDINE** A tight, water-resistant wool form of worsted that has a distinctive diagonal pattern.

▶ **LINEN** An open weave gives linen its ultimate breathability, but wear linen with the knowledge that you'll project a Gatsby-esque bravado—and that within two hours of donning your linen suit you'll be a pile of wrinkles. A linen blazer keeps you cool a bit more neatly.

▶ **TROPICAL** A light wool that is cool and breathable—hence the name—but doesn't hold up as well as worsted.

▶ **TWEED** A fibrous, dense wool that's so warm, a suit of the stuff is overkill on all but the coldest days. As a result, it's more commonly cut into blazers.

▶ **WORSTED** Most suits made from wool are made from worsted. The quality of a worsted is expressed by a number from 120 to 150, which refers to how tightly the individual fibers are twisted. The higher the twist, the smoother, more luxurious, and more expensive the suit will be.

150 **How do I pick a suit pattern?**

It's been said that a truly beautiful man's suit—like a truly handsome face—has to border on the ugly. Some fashionable men's suits have an in-your-face aggressiveness in their stripe, hairiness, or chunky cut. For most occasions, however, a guy needs only an understated elegance, contained in suits that are plain to the point of sobriety.

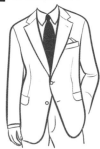

 ▶ **CHALK STRIPES** An evolution on pinstripes that tips the balance more toward bold style than formality. The slightly thicker stripe also adds length to your torso.

 ▶ **GLEN PLAID** Fabric divided neatly by very thin stripes of one or several colors, making for a quietly traditional plaid perfectly suited for spring days and less formal occasions.

 ▶ **HERRINGBONE** Fine chevrons zigzag their way across this pattern, managing to look busy and restrained at the same time. It's possible to carry off a herringbone suit for business. All the same, most herringbone turns up on sport coats, especially ones with leather shooting patches.

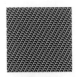

▶ **NAILHEAD** Studded with minuscule dots of a single color, this handsome, conservative pattern is a quiet alternative to solid, and makes it easy to match a tie with the secondary, "nailhead" color.

▶ **PINSTRIPES** These thin stripes, usually of a light color on a dark background, are the businessman's default for good reason: pinstripes give a suit a shot of style without sacrificing an iota of formality. Their complete identification with business, on the other hand, renders them a bit stodgy for social occasions.

▶ **SEERSUCKER** Strictly a warm-weather cotton fabric, this stripe has a happy, Victorian seaside feel. If you want a quieter look than the common blue-and-white palette, go with original "milk and sugar" brown and white.

▶ **SOLID** You can't go wrong with a dark solid-color suit—navy, black, gray, or a green that is very dark and subtle. (Any other colors look like you're going onstage.) Also take into account the occasion: at a wedding, for instance, the bride should be the only one wearing white, and only the band should be wearing a color that outshines the bridesmaids.

151 WHERE SHOULD MY SUIT PANTS BREAK?

WILLIAM BUCKLEY
market editor, *Maxim* magazine

"A lot depends on your age, your height and build, and fashion. We're passing through a period when younger men especially choose no break at all. But it still pays to know how to read that significant crease caused by your cuffs hitting your shoes.

"The classic break occurs two inches above the ankle. It says professional, put together, clean-cut, and is carried best by men of average stature [a]. A full break, barely an inch above the ankle, gives a loose appearance just above the shoes [b]. If worn by the taller man, the full break can look very modern. Shorter men, alas, cannot pull this look off.

"A short break, or even no break at all, is a look that we used to call 'floods' [c]. But with the breakless suit now deemed high fashion, just remember that when you are sitting down, your socks will be defiantly on display. So wear a pair that speaks volumes."

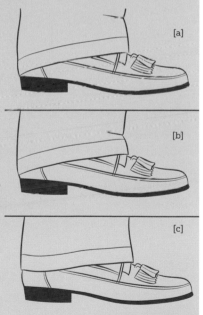

[a]

[b]

[c]

1
2
3
4
5
6

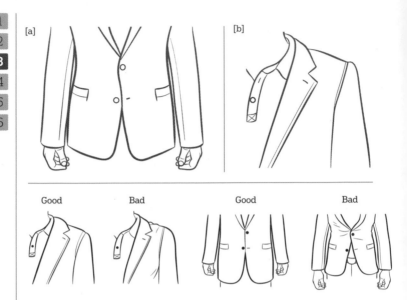

[a] [b]

Good   Bad   Good   Bad

152 How do I know when a jacket fits?

The bottom hem of a suit jacket or sports coat should fall to the first knuckle of your thumb when your arms are at your sides. The sleeve of the jacket should end up somewhere near the base of the wrist—if you like a bit of shirt cuff protruding, go a little longer [a]. The collar should lie flat on the nape of your neck and you should fill out the shoulders and back without being snug [b].

153 How do I take care of a suit?

A tired suit isn't just wrinkled; it's baggy and curly around the lapels. To preserve your suit's sharp lines, don't leave bulky objects like pens or glasses cases in the pockets. Don't crowd it in your closet; suits like a little space to breathe. Otherwise, leave your suit alone. You don't need to have it cleaned after every wearing. Wool naturally repels most of what it encounters in daily wear anyway, and dry cleaning is hard on its fibers. Send a suit to the cleaners after every sixth wearing or so. In the meantime, if it's getting a little wrinkled, hang it in the bathroom with you when you shower and let the steam smooth it out.

154 **Can I wear shorts to work?**

At the office, shorts are an eccentricity that emphasizes the importance of your ideas over your appearance. Fair enough, but like most eccentricities, wearing shorts gives the impression that you represent yourself more than the company—a stance that rarely gets you promoted. If you do throw on shorts for your nine-to-fiver, suppress the urge to wear them with a tie. Outdoor work that doesn't require your legs to be covered for safety's sake invites shorts, of course, but if you're starting a new job, show up on day one in a pair of long work pants.

155 **How often should I shine my shoes?**

Once a week is fine for cleaning up routine wear and tear. If you can't be bothered to do it at home, stop for a shoe shine on the way to work. It makes for a meditative pause at the beginning of your day. While it will set you back $5, it extends the life of the shoe. (Your shoes need regular moisturizing just like you do.)

1
2
3
4
5
6

DIY

156 How do I shine my leather shoes?

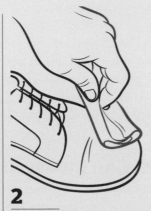

1

Take the shoe trees out of your shoes. (If you don't have shoe trees in, dash out and get a pair. They keep your shoes from curling up at the toes like an elf's.) Untie the laces and loosen them.

2

Wash your shoes—a light rub with a damp cloth will do most days; occasionally you'll want to give them a light bath with clean water. Let any excess water run off and dry them immediately with a rag.

3

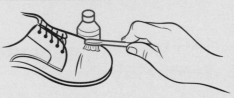

Apply polish or cream in an appropriate color. (Polish is waxier, for protection against water; cream moisturizes the leather. Can't decide? Alternate them each time you shine.) The pros rub the stuff in by hand to work it into the leather's pores, but you can cover your fingers with a cloth. A retired toothbrush will help push the polish into the crease across the front of your shoe and between the upper and sole.

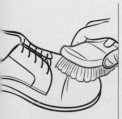

4

After a few minutes, whisk away extra polish with a shoeshine brush. Stand away from your best sheets or your white sofa when you brush, as flecks of polish will fly free. (The bathroom or shower is not a bad place for this step.)

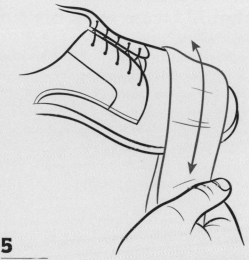

5

Using a soft cotton rag, old T-shirt, chamois, or official buffing cloth, bring up the shine. (Some pros mist the shoes with water before this step.) Hold the cloth by either end and pull it taut against the toe of the shoe and whip it vigorously back and forth, sliding up to the tongue and back down. Moving your hands without losing tension in the rag, buff as much of the upper as the cloth will reach, including the counters at the back of the shoe. Fold the cloth and rub along the sole and up the tongue under the laces.

6

Repeat every two weeks, or about every other time you wear the pair of shoes.

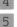

157 Which shoes should I wear with my suit?

Broadly speaking, you have two choices: oxfords and loafers, but within the oxford category alone, you have cap toes, split toes, moc toes, wing tips, and plain. Loafers, meanwhile, extend from schoolboyish penny loafers to chic Italian slippers. (Deck shoes, though technically loafers, are a no-no.) Sneakers, though they occasionally turn up on cheeky filmmakers and guys with foot maladies, should not be worn with suits.

Lace-up boots are acceptable, too, and if the material of your suit is heavy enough, like tweed, you can strike a countryman's figure with a low-cut, dark work boot, especially if the cut is full and your pants are cuffed, but not at work.

Black shoes can be worn with navy and gray; brown and cordovan shoes go with anything brown or tan, of course, as well as gray and even navy if they are dark.

158 How do I know which tie to wear?

The array of ties in the menswear section of a department store can be overwhelming. Here is a guide to a few of the different types and what they will say about you.

▶ **FLOWER POWER** The '80s popularity of Liberty of London's pretty floral patterns liberated men to expand into feminine but attractive options, like the tie designs of Vineyard Vines, which carry even more insider cachet.

▶ **GOOFY TIES** What hangs around a man's neck is one of the few places in an otherwise closely restricted wardrobe where a man can be frivolous. That said, be conscious that a tie decorated with cartoon characters, sports insignia, or anything related to golf—unless you work for ESPN—says "I'd rather be elsewhere." Absolutely avoid photography and pornography.

▶ **POWER TIES** In the beginning there was the IBM salesman's *de rigueur* red tie. Then, after the lawlessness of the 1970s, yellow ties reigned on VIP necks for most of the 1980s. Now every few years, the standard-bearers of business fashion anoint a new color as the power hue. Regis made ties that matched his shirts popular, and Donald Trump has made pink ties hip. Watch the neckwear of key figures like the treasury secretary and lawyers leaving courthouses with high-powered clients.

▶ **REP TIES** Based on the striped ties of Britain's public-school uniforms, rep (sometimes "repp") ties still summon a schoolboyish charm, but are also useful in introducing several colors into a given day's ensemble, making it easier to match to your suit or shirt.

159 **How do I know which knot to use?**

First, consider your collar. Spread collars tend to look better with a fatter knot, like a Windsor or half Windsor, while pointed collars look best with the four-in-hand. But you don't have to be ruled by your collar choice. A four-in-hand, even on a spread collar, implies subtlety and depth of thought. The half Windsor, whose chunky shape exudes

1
2
3
4
5
6

confidence, works well for job interviews. The full Windsor, a power statement, can be a little obnoxious when worn using a thick, shiny tie, but if you want to rule the roost, it's the only choice.

160 **How do I tie a half-Windsor knot?**

With the tie over your neck, pull the wide end of the tie down until its point touches your pants' zipper flap [a]. The long end will now be your action end. Cross it over the short end, and bring it back over the crossing [b]. Tug it to your left before looping it under the crossing point and up again in front of the burgeoning knot. The long end will now have its seam showing front [c]. Flip it to your right again, go behind the knot and over [d]. Thread the point carefully through the

HALF WINDSOR

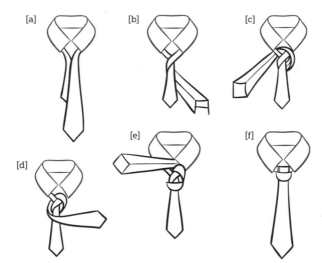

[a] [b] [c]

[d] [e] [f]

outside loop of the knot [e]. Tug it gently downward until the tie tightens [f]. Now lightly grasp the short end with a thumb and forefinger as you press the knot into place with your other hand.

161 **How do I tie a four-in-hand?**

Start with the tie draped over your neck, seam side in, with the wide end several inches below your belt buckle [a]. Cross the wide end over the narrow end [b], then flip the wide end over again and bring the point of the wide end up [c], passing it behind the burgeoning knot and over. As you bring it down, pass the point of the wide end through the last loop you made at the front of the knot [d]. Tug the wide end down gently [e] and push the knot up as in the half Windsor [f].

FOUR-IN-HAND

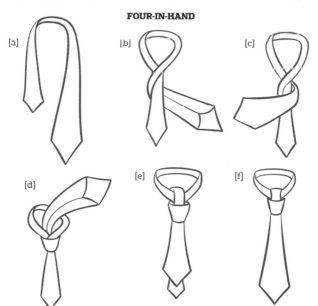

[a] [b] [c]

[d] [e] [f]

162 **When should I wear a bow tie?**

A bow tie is de rigueur when wearing a traditional tux or dinner jacket, and is useful whenever you don't want your full tie interfering with your work. (This is why waiters, gas-station attendants, and photographers stereotypically wore bow ties.)

But depending on color and pattern, the bow tie runs the style gamut from dandyish to southern gentleman to professorial. As long as you sport its slightly outdated look with confidence, the bow tie's use needn't be restricted by occasion or the rest of your outfit: a suit takes a bow tie as well as a blazer. Note: a bow tie tied by hand always looks better than a clip-on.

GUYS' LIST

Ten novels every guy should read

▶ *THE GREAT GATSBY*
F. Scott Fitzgerald (1925)

▶ *THE SUN ALSO RISES*
Ernest Hemingway (1926)

▶ *THE MALTESE FALCON*
Dashiell Hammett (1930)

▶ *INVISIBLE MAN*
Ralph Ellison (1952)

▶ *RABBIT, RUN*
John Updike (1960)

▶ *CATCH-22*
Joseph Heller (1961)

▶ *PORTNOY'S COMPLAINT*
Philip Roth (1969)

▶ *SLAUGHTERHOUSE-FIVE*
Kurt Vonnegut (1969)

▶ *THE SPORTSWRITER*
Richard Ford (1986)

▶ *THE THINGS THEY CARRIED*
Tim O'Brien (1990)

163 **How do I tie a bow tie?**

You'll be relieved to know that a bow tie doesn't have to be as perfect as those ready-made ones you get with your rental tux. A real bow tie should be tight, but have a slightly disheveled rakishness.

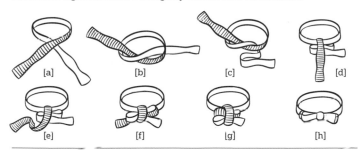

[a]   [b]   [c]   [d]

[e]   [f]   [g]   [h]

1

Let the tie hang so that the left end is slightly longer than the other [a]. Begin like you're tying a shoe, crossing the longer end over the shorter and tucking it up and over the short end [b]. Flip that longer end back over your shoulder for the time being [c].

2

Fold the shorter end into a bow-tie shape and hold it against your collar button [d]. Don't let go of this bow for the rest of the process.

3

Let the longer end fall from your shoulder [e]. Place your forefinger in its center and push it through the loop behind the bow you're holding against your collar [f]. As it passes through the hole, the longer end will fold into a second bow [g]. Make sure both folded ends are on opposite sides of the tie.

4

Gently pull the bow tight, and fiddle with the ends and bows until the tie is as orderly as you like [h].

1
2
3
4
5
6

164 **How do I dress for casual days?**

Casual doesn't mean you have to leave your style at home with your suits. Denim gives you a dark-on-bottom look that will set you apart from the khaki crowd. Top your jeans off with a dress shirt in a trim cut, and give the look a strong base with lace-up ankle boots, side buckles, or even the wing tips or cap toes you wear with your suits—anything, that is, but Topsiders unless you're going for a retro-preppy look.

WHEN BUSINESS MEETS PLEASURE

165 **How do I act at a business lunch?**

A business lunch is part of your work life. Though the point is to get off-site and relax, your behavior reflects on your potential as a colleague or partner. Treat the restaurant staff as you would ideally treat colleagues: it will be taken as a measure of how you'll be to work with and how you'll represent the firm.

Order lightly, even if you have to grab a snack before you meet. The point of the meal is business, not satisfying your appetite. (Your dining companion may also view your restraint as an indication of how you'll deal with his or her budget or your expense account.)

Stick with simple dishes that won't claim your attention. Stay away from pasta dishes dripping with sauce that requires maximum dipping and slurping. And if you expect the meeting to get tense, don't order spicy food that will saw holes in your already acid stomach.

166 How do I deal with romantic advances from the boss?

A guy is loath to turn down sex from any quarter, but taking part in sexy talk and accepting invitations, especially from a superior, could put your job in danger. Even if the encounter leaves the two of you as friends, your hot action is a liability for the company, and if anyone finds out, both your jobs are likely toast. It may be that you and your boss are feeling a deepening love as you work together; invite her to have a serious discussion outside work about the future of the relationship. If the advances are unwelcome, make it plain to the boss, and inform a colleague (whom you trust) the first time it happens, to serve as a witness should you need one. The second time, report the person to HR.

167 Should I friend my boss online?

The boss may well be overjoyed to have any employee reach out to him or her, but given your unequal relationship, protocol dictates that you should wait for your boss to make the request. Accept immediately. The Internet has opened up new doors for professional networking, and friending the boss will open you to all his contacts. Just make sure your privacy settings are up and running so when your goofy college roommate thinks it's funny to post old photos the boss is sufficiently screened.

168 **How do I have private conversations at work?**

Never talk where you can't see who is listening. People have been fired by a booming voice from a toilet stall. If you have to speak to a colleague privately, find an empty office or a conference room and have your chat there. Or if that's not possible, see if you can take your chat outside—take a walk around the block or grab a coffee.

Communicating verbally is by far the safest method. Don't write any confidential matters or gossip in e-mail. Once you send an e-mail, you lose control over who can read your words. The same applies to IM and even personal e-mail. Your company has the right to anything and everything you do on your work computers, laptops, and desktops alike. Use the phone or face-to-face conversation to tell all secrets.

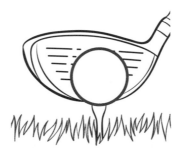

169 **What are the rules for playing golf for business?**

Golf has become an adjunct to the office for many guys. Salesmen cement relationships on the course, while lawyers, bankers, and brokers take clients out to thank them for past business in the hope of more in the future. A few ground rules for making golf work for you:

▶ **DON'T LET BUSINESS DOMINATE** The whole ritual collapses if the guy you invited realizes that you invited him to play golf only to hound him for business. Wait for your guest to initiate business conversation and provide a concise response or suggest somebody at your firm who can provide assistance. Then hit the ball, or tell a joke, but don't spend the remainder of the hole expanding on your answer. Wait for your guest to ask another question.

▶ **PLAY AT HOME** If you invite someone golfing, have tee times reserved someplace where you play routinely—hopefully where somebody, if not every valet parker, locker-room guy, golf pro, and starter knows you by name.

▶ **PAY TO PLAY** As host, you pick up the tab from the moment your companions' feet hit the parking lot to the moment they leave: greens fees, tips, lunch, and beverages—everything but their souvenir hat or shirt—is on you.

▶ **MATCH PLAY** Dial back your game if you're better than the client, and comment self-deprecatingly if he's better than you. If possible, find out if your guest has a registered handicap with the USGA. Only serious golfers have handicaps. It's best if you are at the same talent level, since your competitive juices will start to flow. The client will remember the game fondly and you'll have that positive memory to work from.

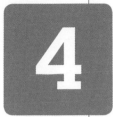

4

Skills

No man is born knowing how to change a tire or play
poker. The skills needed to get through life are the
product of experience and a few handy tips.
Here are some to get you started.

CHORES, REPAIRS, AND FIX-UPS

170 **How do I paint a room?**

It takes time to do the job right—budget at least a day to do an average-size room between all of the preparations and the different coats—but few household improvements are as satisfying as the neatly painted room you did yourself.

▶ **PREP** Move the furniture to the center of the room and cover it with sheet plastic. Lay painter's paper on the floor and tape it in place. Put masking tape over exposed horizontal surfaces, like windowsills and the tops of floorboards. With a putty knife, scrape off loose paint. Fill any holes with joint compound by putting a small amount on the leading edge of a putty knife and smoothing it into the cracks. Allow to dry, and rub or sand the spot until it's perfectly even with the wall or ceiling. Paint water stains and other discolored spots with a sealer.

▶ **PRIME** Starting at the end of the room with the most light, "cut in" the ceiling by painting a straight, two- or three-inch line around its edge, then roll the paint onto the remaining area. Roll the shortest distance across the ceiling, not lengthwise, occasionally rolling at an angle to cover nicely but always finishing with a straight stroke. Do everything you can to reach from one place before moving your ladder. While the ceiling dries, paint the walls, cutting in at the corners and rolling the rest.

▶ **COLOR** Apply the first coat of the ceiling and wall color by the same process. When you come to the end of a wall, make sure you have enough paint in the open can for the entire next wall. If you don't, mix in more paint from another can and stir; beginning a new can in the middle of a wall may result in a visible change in shade. When the entire room is dry, add a second coat.

171 **How do I measure to cut a piece of wood?**

The soul of good carpentry, accurate measuring consists of two skills: developing an eye for the tape measure's calibrations, and marking your measurements properly.

To measure properly you need to get familiar with the tape measure—there are so many lines of differing heights that sometimes you can't see the forest for the trees. It's about training your eye to spot measurements rapidly, not about the math. Begin by fixing on one line as your handy reference point: five-eighths is a good one because it's sufficiently precise—a lot of measurements you'll make will require you to think in eighths and sixteenths, not the relatively chunky fourths. Once your eye gets accustomed to seeing the five-eighths line, it's easy to drill down to sixteenths.

Never measure without a pencil in your hand, and mark your measurements without letting diagonals sneak in. If you're cutting a piece of plywood, measure along the top edge, make a mark and then measure and mark the bottom. Connect the two marks using a straightedge. On lumber, don't use a simple line, which can wobble. Draw a V-shape (called "crow's feet") on either side of the point you're measuring to, so you know exactly where to cut.

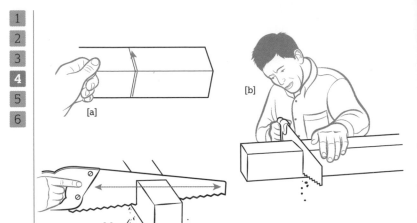

172 **How do I use a saw?**

Making sure your wood is steady, place the saw's blade to the outer side of your mark [a]. (If you cut directly on the mark, your cut will be off by the width of the saw's blade, about one-sixth of an inch.) Saw using the entire length of the blade and take your time, letting the saw's teeth do the work [b]. Putting too much pressure on the blade gives you a ragged cut and makes a hash of the saw's edge [c].

173 **What's the secret to a perfectly mowed lawn?**

A weekly clipping keeps grass looking neater and feeling thicker. Mow in a pattern: straight lines, circles, or imitating the helmet logo of your football team—it doesn't matter as long as you remember what you did last time and alter the pattern week to week to keep your grass "honest": constant grooming in one direction causes the grass to lie flat and duck the mower blades. To mow in straight lines, use the sidewalk or curb, if any, as a straightedge. Overlap your last course across the lawn by the width of the mower's tire so you don't end up with uncut strays. Look for swales—low spots in the ground—and mow these from several angles to make sure your mower blades reach all the grass.

174 **How do I keep my grass green?**

Grass naturally turns brown about late June—after which, that lush color has to be propped up with a little chemistry. Hit the lawn with a slow-release nitrogen mix twice in late spring and twice in the fall—a good plan for the middle of the United States is mid-April, mid-June, and late September or early October. (If you mulch your nitrogen-rich grass clippings instead of bagging them, you can cut back on the amount of fertilizer you put down by a quarter.)

Grass also goes dormant, and brown, when it gets dehydrated. Mow your grass toward evening or just before it rains, and leave the grass at least two inches high, especially in the hottest months. And get the hose out weekly to give it a deep soak.

The better your lawn looks, one should note, the worse it is for the environment. Rather than struggle to sustain grass for a whole hot season, you can do yourself and the planet a favor and plant a mix of grass, clover, herbs, and wildflowers. Available at garden stores and online, these mixes look a bit eccentric until you and the neighbors get used to it, but it will stand up to serious heat and foot traffic without much water or fertilizer. Pure clover is another eco-friendly, though somewhat fragile, possibility, or dispense with lawn management altogether by planting moss, or a creeping vine like English ivy.

1
2
3
4
5
6

DIY

175 How do I sew a button on a shirt?

1

Pick up a simple sewing kit at any pharmacy, which should come with needles and a set of different colored threads. Make sure you pick the right-size needle. For a shirt button you'll want the medium-size regular needle.

2

Check the other buttons to see how they are sewn on. You'll imitate this pattern.

3

Unspool two feet of thread, using the same color as the other buttons. Insert one end through the eye of a needle (a little moisture and a twist on the thread helps). Bring the ends together so the needle hangs from the thread's midpoint. Tie the ends together with a small knot.

4

Moving from inside the shirt out, take your thread through the spot where you want the button to sit and then sew through the button's holes in the same pattern as all the other buttons. Pull the knot snug each time, but not so snug that you won't be able to maneuver the button once you're finished.

5

Continue the accustomed pattern until you have about four inches of thread left and the needle is inside the shirt.

6

Free the needle with a snip of your scissors and tie a knot snug to the fabric, then another, landing it as close to the first as you can. Snip off the thread a half inch or so from the second knot.

176 How do I grow grass from seed?

In the first weeks of summer, prepare the soil by breaking up clods, removing stones and rival growth with a heavy-tined garden rake. Mix in topsoil and compost as you go. Have on hand a seed that suits the climate—bluegrass, fescue, and ryegrass in the Northeast, Bermuda where it's warmer—and the amount of shade present at midday. Sow the seed by hand, hurling the seed down so it embeds itself nicely in the soil. Don't blanket the soil completely—a seed every half inch or so will do the trick. With your seed down, distribute a fluffy, spare layer of sphagnum or peat moss over the seed and water immediately.

Your seed needs you most now. Continue watering religiously for five days, soaking the ground in the morning and at dusk until the water is just beginning to stand on the soil. For another week, make sure to water at least once a day. In a week to ten days, you'll see the first fuzz of green. Keep the water coming, but don't mow until the grass is thickening on its own, about four weeks later.

177 Is there a good technique for pruning bushes and shrubs?

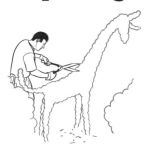

You have two basic types of bushes in your yard: hedges and ornamental shrubs. Hedges, like privet or boxwood, should be trimmed a few times each summer in order to maintain a neat look. For creating the flat sides and sharp edges of hedges or a solid orb of an evergreen bush, an electric clipper is ideal.

Hedges and other solid bushes should be cut back to their desired shape in the spring as they get ready for their main growth spurt of the year. But each species of hedge or shrub needs to be cut with an understanding of its growing habits. Some evergreens, like euonymus, are fast growers and will come back quickly from a "hard cut"; others, like hemlock, should be trimmed only a few inches. Before you prune anything, get to know the growth habits of the plants in your yard and make a plan.

When cutting ornamental shrubs, avoid solid shapes. When trimming ornamental shrubs like lilac, azalea, forsythia, or andromeda, use a hand pruner to preserve the plant's natural, open shape. Flowering shrubs should not be cut before they flower, nor too late in the year, when they are setting bud for the following season. Instead, trim flowering shrubs between their bloom and late July. To thicken the shrub, clip back any whips that have shot out more than four inches and clip inside the bush to make the interior branches split in two.

178 **What's the foolproof way to do laundry?**

Nobody likes doing laundry, but if you do a load every week, the task won't be so daunting next time you tackle it.

▶ **SORT** Dump your dirties onto an open space on the floor and deal them into piles by color: dark colors like green, black, and dark blue here; reds and pinks there; whites in another pile; and "lights," a fungible category that stretches from light blues to khaki. You don't want to overstuff a washing machine, so if any pile amounts to more than you can carry between navel and collarbone between your two arms, break it into two piles.

▶ **READ** Manufacturers are required to inform you how to wash their garments. If something's new, find a tag bearing instructions, no matter how well they've hidden it, and segregate the item accordingly into piles to dry-clean, hand-wash, or wash cold or warm. Dry-clean only goes to the dry cleaner, of course; hand-wash only you'll have to take care of in the sink with a little bit of detergent and some elbow grease; the cold- and warm-wash piles you'll separate and stick into the machine.

▶ **FILL** A washing machine has three basic options: temperature of the washing water, size of the load, and vigor/duration of wash. You've got the first two sorted already. As for vigor, most things can handle the regular cycle; woolens and other colds appreciate a delicate cycle, which often asks you to set the duration of wash. Go for the full ride.

Detergent should be added before you load in the clothes. Look for a small door outside the washer or just inside the machine's lid marked "detergent," which, when the water runs in, mixes the soap with the water automatically. Otherwise, dump the soap straight in. Let the detergent lather half a minute or so. Put your clothes in and shut the top to the washer.

▶ **DRY** After the last spin, toss your load into the dryer. (At the Laundromat, look for a dryer that has been recently in use, to capitalize on the already warm drum.) The machine may give you the option of normal drying and a more gentle cycle. Normal is fine for everything except wool items, which will shrink in heat; hang them from your shower rod on hangers.

▶ **FOLD** To avoid wrinkles, fold everything as soon as it comes out of the dryer. And then you're done!

179 **How do I iron a shirt?**

Set the iron at the hottest temperature your fabric will allow. Most irons' temperature gauge includes a guide. For cotton shirts, use the cotton setting. An iron with a spray function is desirable, or use a plastic spray bottle (like the ones designed for houseplants) to mist your shirt as you iron.

Turn your shirt inside out, to protect it from the iron, and lay the collar on the ironing board facedown. Moving in an easy zigzag motion forward and back, press the collar against the ironing board in two passes: once lightly to spread the fabric flat against the board's surface, then applying greater pressure once you're confident you won't be ironing wrinkles into it [a].

Insert the point of the ironing board into the shirt's armhole until the shoulder and upper sleeve are stretched flat [b]. Iron that area, then turn the shirt and arrange one side of the shirtfront on the board [c]. Iron from the top down, using the iron's narrow end to negotiate around the buttons. Turn the shirt on the board until you've gone around the sides, back, and the opposite front panel [d].

If your shirt has a placket—that extra layer of cloth running down the buttonhole edge—turn the shirt right side out and carefully run the iron, pointed edge first, back up the placket from the outside.

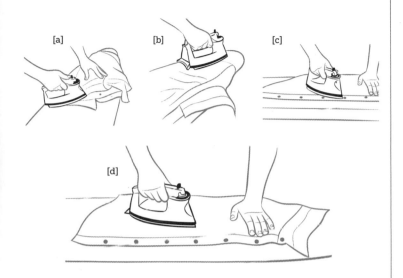

[a] [b] [c] [d]

On the same panel may be a breast pocket. Iron that on the outside side as well. Last, lay each sleeve out flat in turn and iron it.

You can iron ties, too, but carefully. With the iron on a low setting, lay the tie flat, facedown on the ironing board, and cover the part that needs to be pressed with a thick towel. Iron through the towel. If, after a few passes, the wrinkles are still there, bump up the heat a little until they are gone.

180 **What are the rules when house-sitting?**

You're doing your pal a favor by looking out for his dog, his plants, or just maintaining a human presence while he's gone, but behave as you would expect a good houseguest should. If he's got a monster TV and a king-size bed, let him know you're going to put both to optimum use and be respectful doing so; if it's a monk's cell, point out that you need some time to catch up on work, or reading, away from distractions. He should go away feeling that his house is as highly valued, and therefore as safe, as when he's home.

Get to the place a day or two before the start of your sit, to go through the checklist of what needs to be done each day. Make sure you have a full set of keys and try them out to make sure you know which is which. Ask your pal to introduce you to at least one neighbor who can vouch that you're legit in case someone contests your comings and goings. Establish how he'd like you to deal with phone calls (answer or let the machine pick up everything?) and get an itinerary from your pal so you know where to reach him in case of emergencies.

Once you take possession of the place, keep things orderly, don't have more than one or two guests at a time, and disturb as little of his personal stuff as possible. It's okay to move a piece of furniture or clear off a desk temporarily if you need a space to work or do sit-ups, but in general live as if you expected him to walk in any minute—which he might.

On the day of his scheduled arrival, remake the bed with clean sheets, clean out the fridge, water the plants, and make the place at least as welcoming and tidy as the day he left. Being a gracious guest is one way to ensure you'll be invited to housesit again.

181 **How do I babysit?**

Offering (or complying with a request) to babysit a strapped friend's kid is one of the most valorous duties you can perform. It's often as simple as taking the sprite to the movies, or to a cheesy meal—literally, since pizza or cheeseburgers with fries will make you a hero.

(Be sure to check with Mom and Dad about any food allergies first.) If you're housebound, overplan the time; bring an activity or board game you'd like to try, and a video.

Don't be shy about laying down the law. Every adult has the responsibility to instruct children, just as every adult has the responsibility to treat kids with respect. Call the kid out on behavior that is not appropriate, and try to engage the child in another activity. Never grab a child unless they are about to do bodily harm to themselves or another person, including you, but feel free to pick up a toddler to redirect him from a situation.

182 Holding a baby freaks me out—how do I do it properly?

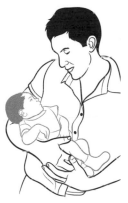

If it's your first time, it's probably best to sit down. Fold your arms loosely in front of you, lift one elbow slightly away from your body, and slide your opposite hand beneath it. As you take the baby, rest its head in the crook of the elbow, while you support his or her back with your hand. When you feel comfortable, don't be afraid to stand up and walk with the child in your arms.

183 Can I fix my computer myself?

No matter how oddly it's behaving, or what you stupidly stuck into it, thousands of computers are doing the *exact same thing*. Before you take it to a pro, confess your problem to your favorite search engine

EXPERT WITNESS

184 HOW DO I KEEP PAPERWORK FROM PILING UP?

CARLA KOEHL
founder of Plan A, an organizing and design company

"Divide your papers into two piles, the filing pile and the next-action pile. File away anything that you've completed from your records, but note: nothing goes into a file until it requires no more action. Everything in your next-action pile goes into your calendar. If there's no firm deadline for action, make an actual date when you're going to make a decision. Or pick one item and give yourself an hour to make a decision. If it's a longer-term thing, divide it into steps and keep benchmarks along the way. Force yourself to make a decision."

and see what your fellow sufferers have to say. Check the manufacturer's site, too: you may find that so many thousands have the same complaint that an extended warranty has been offered.

185 How many computer passwords should I have?

Ideally you should have as many passwords as you have logins, but in practice, this invites chaos. Devise a few strong passwords and never use the same password for two sites in the same category: online banking, credit cards, or other financial instruments should each have their own, as should your social networks and your work and home computers.

FIELD, WOODS, AND HIGHWAY

186 **How do I throw a perfect spiral?**

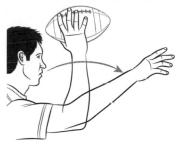

Hold the ball as far back on the laces as you need to get a tight grip. As you bring your arm forward, your wrist should be cocked backward ninety degrees. As your hand and the ball pass just behind and above your ear, straighten your wrist with a snap so your hand ends up palm down. Follow through with your arm until your fingers are pointed directly at the ground.

187 **How do I nail a runner at the plate?**

It helps to have a gun for an arm, but a little technique goes a long way. Grasp the ball toward the ends of your first two fingers, perpendicular to the red stitches and with your fingertips firmly planted on the stitches. Position your thumb on the opposite side of the ball from, and in line with, your index finger. With your arm aloft in an L-shape, cock your wrist backward toward your elbow so that the ball is about even with your ear.

Point your front-facing shoulder directly to your target. Step forward abruptly as you bring the arm holding the ball sharply over

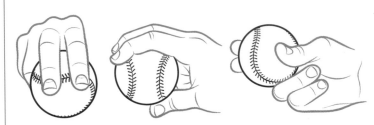

Fingers go on the stitches

your head in a straight-up-and-down arc. Uncock your wrist with a snap as you let the ball fly so the ball rotates backward toward you in flight. (This will give the ball extra loft.) Follow through, bringing your arm across your body until your throwing hand is nearly touching the opposite knee.

188 **How do I train for a marathon?**

Pick your first marathon for its scenic beauty and its size—a medium-to-large event with anywhere from ten thousand to forty thousand runners will probably be better organized and more exciting than a local race. Most important, have a goal: the mental part of marathoning is critical, and when you hit the wall in those last six miles, you'll need to focus on why you wanted to put yourself through this misery. Some people run for charities or in remembrance of a loved one. Maybe you run just to say you've done it but having a higher purpose can help.

Mark the date on your calendar and start training about twenty weeks out. For the first few weeks, just get comfortable running. Find your best pace and maintain it for at least a half hour. Then with six-teen weeks to go, switch to a mileage regimen roughly like this:

MARATHON MILE TRAINING

WEEK	DAY 1	DAY 2	DAY 3	DAY 4	TOTAL
1	3	4	3	5	**15**
2	3	4	3	6	**16**
3	3	4	3	7	**17**
4	3	5	3	8	**19**
5	3	5	3	10	**21**
6	4	5	4	11	**24**
7	4	6	4	12	**26**
8	4	6	4	14	**28**
9	4	7	4	16	**31**
10	5	8	5	16	**34**
11	5	8	5	17	**35**
12	5	8	5	18	**36**
13	5	8	5	20	**38**
14	5	8	5	9	**27**
15	3	5	3	8	**19**

The last days before the marathon, taper off further, running only three miles or so a day to let your legs recover from training. The day before the race, walk a couple of miles, but mostly rest.

189 Should I drink water or energy drinks while exercising?

A big glass of water anywhere from an hour to a half hour before you exert yourself, then another H_2O dose when you finish should hold you for any amount of exercise up to an hour. After that, your body starts to look for something to replace the minerals that help your system run. At about the sixty-minute mark, restore your electrolytes with an energy drink, an energy bar, or some energy goo—a gel packed with carbs and electrolytes.

1
2
3
4
5
6

Whatever energy booster you choose, don't drink or swallow anything for the first time in the middle of an important workout. As with new shoes or shorts, you shouldn't find out how your body likes something new on a race day.

190 **What can I do to run faster?**

The more times your foot hits the ground in the course of a race, the faster you go. This is how a short-legged runner can defeat a long-legged one: he steps at a higher tempo. Measure your own tempo by running for thirty seconds, counting the number of steps you take. Now run thirty seconds back, increasing the number of steps you take without limiting the length of your stride. You can also reset your running tempo by gunning hard downhill, then keeping the same pace as you hit level ground. Once you find a sustainable fast pace, mix a short run of twenty minutes or so in which you run as hard as you can into your usual regimen.

191 **How do I win a footrace?**

Stay with the pack, letting the front-runners find (and eventually lose) their legs. As you run, identify the best runners, the guys with loping but rapid strides. They, like you, will be biding their time just behind the front-runners. As you come to the last quarter of the race, grab the lead without announcing your move with foot slaps or grunting. Once you're in front, stay there. Strictly maintain the most direct route to the finish so your competitors will have to go around you to finish. Their extra steps should provide you the edge you need to win.

192 What do I wear on a hike?

So long as he's in civilization, a guy should wear natural fibers. Beyond its borders, space-age synthetics wick the moisture away from your skin, keeping you drier. Synthetics also retain body heat better when you get drenched by the elements. A couple of tight-fitting polyester T-shirts and an acrylic hat are an excellent investment. In cold weather, top off with a layer of wool.

193 What should I bring on a day hike?

Bring lots of water, a high-carb snack (a traditional hiker's food is "gorp": a mix of granola, raisins, peanuts, and sometimes chocolate chips); a light rain jacket that fits over a synthetic fleece; and a hat. Even if you don't plan on being out after dark, an emergency blanket and a flashlight will make you feel very smart if something goes wrong.

194 What do I need for walking on the trail?

Don't put a forty-pound bag on your back the first day and think you're going to walk ten miles. Pack your bag a few weeks ahead—you'll want to do this to practice fitting all your gear inside anyway—and build up your stamina by walking around the block, then a mile, then a few miles. Or walk five miles a day over a period of time, adding more weight to your bag each time out. Remember to stretch before and after each workout.

195 How can I start a fire without matches?

You probably know you can use a magnifying glass, but any lens or something that can be polished or manipulated to produce halos of intense light will do: eyeglasses, ice, a baggy, even a condom. Gather very dry, wispy organic stuff like dead tall grass and leaves— a lot of it, since once lit, it will have to light longer-burning material, like dry twigs, which you should also collect in advance. Concentrate the light on your tinder, moving it from one inch to two inches away until the light's edges are not fuzzy. The thinnest tendrils of your stuff will soon ignite.

No condom, ice, or magnifying glass? (What *do* you bring?) With your tinder collected, make an indentation in a flat piece of wood with a knife [a]. Peel the bark from a two-foot-long stick and place it beside the indentation. Rest the stick in the indentation and swivel it rapidly between your hands, bearing down on the tip and keeping your soon-to-be-forming sweat away from

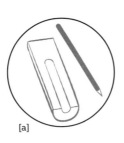

[a]

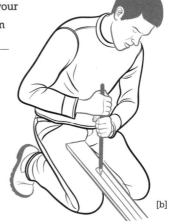

[b]

the tip [b]. Don't give up. Eventually a tiny ember will appear, which you can shove onto your bark, then scrape onto your flammable pile. Blow gently until it ignites.

196 **How do I find north during the day?**

Find a straight stick and insert it upright in the ground [a]. Mark the length of the shadow and then mark again in ten to fifteen minutes [b]. Draw a straight line between the two marks. This is roughly your east–west line with your second mark at the eastern end. If you stand with the west marker on your left and the east on your right, you are most likely facing north [c].

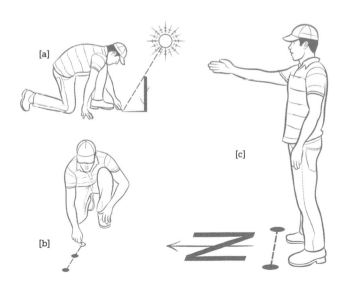

1
2
3
4
5
6

197 **How do I find north at night?**

Find a particularly bright star and sit down with a stick. Hold the stick so you are looking along the length of it at the star. Bracing your elbows against your rib cage for stability, keep looking for a few minutes. If the star has moved to the left of your stick, you're facing north. If it has moved right, you're facing south. If up, east; down, west.

198 **What do I need to sleep outdoors?**

You'll need a tent if the weather is particularly wet, cold, or both. But tents are only a starting point. You'll need a sleeping bag with synthetic fill that will retain its insulating qualities when wet, and a foam pad that buffers the cold as well as the hardness of the ground. In warm weather, you can get away with your sleeping bag and foam pad and a tarp with grommets at the edges and a few tent stakes. An eight-by-ten tarp is lighter than all but the priciest tents, and offers many modes of shelter: a canopy hung over a ridge line, a lean-to, or a flat roof suspended by all four corners.

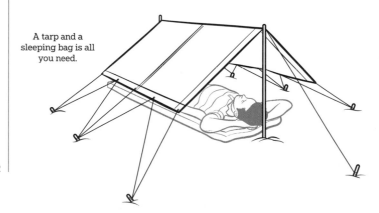

A tarp and a sleeping bag is all you need.

Note: when picking out a tent, add one person to the advertised capacity. A one-person tent will accommodate you, barely, but not your backpack.

199 What should I eat to prepare for a big day of exercise?

Start the night before with a large meal full of carbohydrates, fats, and protein—spaghetti with meatballs or beef Stroganoff over egg noodles. A beer or two, especially a dark ale or lager, won't hurt either, as long as you drink water to stay hydrated. In the morning, go lighter, but get the same combination of food groups: oatmeal with nuts and wheat germ, a cheese omelet with sausage, or pancakes with bacon. These slow-burning calories will fuel a long day of exertion.

200 What should I eat on the trail?

For a single-night excursion, this is a no-brainer: steak (packed in an icy pouch), wine, and potatoes, with a hank of foil for baking them in the fire's embers. But when you're solo or on a multiday hike, you need food that is light and nutritious, in serious amounts. These foods should keep you going throughout the day.

▶ **BAGELS** Whole-wheat bagels won't get squished or broken like sliced bread, and often smuggle in more protein.

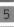

DIY

201 What can I use to make my own cookstove?

Some trail experts don't carry an expensive, heavy stove with them; they substitute a bottle of rubbing alcohol and a soda or other metal can. Here's how:

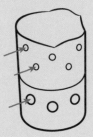

Tuna

1

Find an old soda can. Cut out the top with your knife.

2

Cut holes about one inch from the bottom and two offset rows of holes near the top.

▶ **NUTS, DRIED FRUIT, SUNFLOWER SEEDS** Keep a supply of these no-water-weight snacks on hand during the day to keep your fuel needle from dropping too far.

▶ **TUNA IN OIL** Ounce for ounce, the most durable, satisfying, and adaptable protein-and-fat combo available, even when you count the heavy can, which, anyway, you can convert to a cookstove in a pinch (see above).

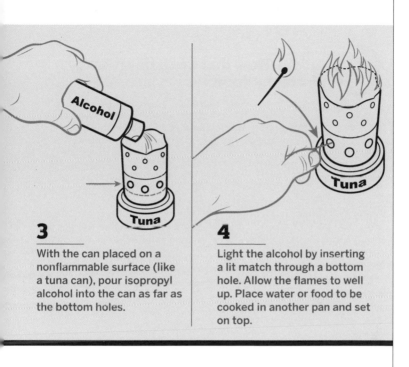

3

With the can placed on a nonflammable surface (like a tuna can), pour isopropyl alcohol into the can as far as the bottom holes.

4

Light the alcohol by inserting a lit match through a bottom hole. Allow the flames to well up. Place water or food to be cooked in another pan and set on top.

▶ **DRY RAMEN NOODLES** Good for stoking up on carbs, and lighter than bread.

▶ **RICE AND DRIED BEANS** A simple, balanced protein-and-carb meal, these staples, even in quantity, won't weigh you down. As you walk, soak that night's portion of beans in a plastic bag suspended from your backpack or else secured in a watertight container in your pack. When you're ready to eat, they'll soften in less than an hour of boiling.

1
2
3
4
5
6

202 **How do I keep bears away from my food?**

Bears gave their name to the simple contraption called a bear hang, but it's as effective in deterring—and probably more often serves to deter—raccoons, skunks, and squirrels.

1

Find two trees not too far apart with their lowest branches about fifteen feet from the ground. If you have heard that there are bears in the area, the trees should be no closer than a hundred feet from your tent, and the branches should not be strong enough to support a young bear.

2

Tie a weight like a rock to one end of a rope and toss it over one branch.

3

Pack all your comestibles and anything with a pleasing scent—soap, toothpaste, sunblock, and deodorant—into two sacks.

4

Tie the rope around the neck of one sack and hoist it into the air. Do the same with the other sack, tucking any loose rope into the sack. Push the second sack upward with a stick until both sacks are about twelve feet off the ground. Make sure you have a stick long enough to pull the sacks down again in the morning.

203 **Which knots should I know?**

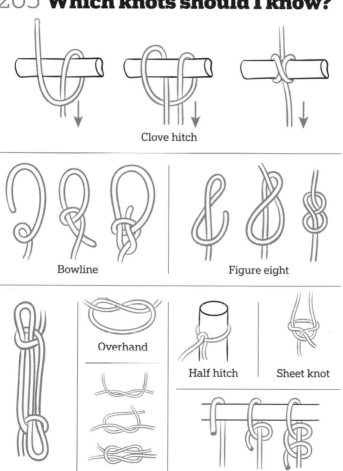

Clove hitch

Bowline

Figure eight

Overhand

Half hitch

Sheet knot

Sheepshank

Reef knot

Two half hitches

1
2
3
4
5
6

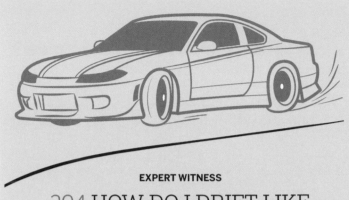

EXPERT WITNESS

204 HOW DO I DRIFT LIKE THEY DO IN *THE FAST AND THE FURIOUS*?

SAMUEL HUBINETTE
Formula Drift champion and stunt driver on
The Fast and the Furious: Tokyo Drift

"Accelerate first. If you have a clutch, rev your engine and release the clutch really quick. Otherwise, shift the weight of the vehicle over its wheels—we call this method 'load transfer'—by turning to the left and then quickly to the right. You want to flick the car to one side and back to the other. You'll feel the drift begin in the direction your wheel is turned.

"Once you start to drift, control your skid with your power. Add more throttle to increase the angle, back off the accelerator to straighten out. Make sure you have lots of room to execute your drift—try a big parking lot or a racetrack. Once you get the hang of it, practice by drifting in circles around a safety cone."

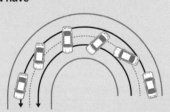

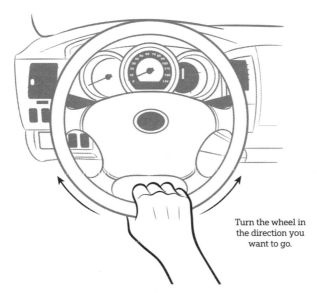

Turn the wheel in the direction you want to go.

205 **How do I back up a trailer?**

Driving in reverse requires your brain to flip its usual hand-eye directions, a puzzle complicated further when you have another wheeled vehicle attached by a hitch at your bumper. Simplify the process by putting one hand at the bottom of the steering wheel. As you back up, move your hand in the direction you want the trailer to go: up to the left to turn the trailer leftward out of a driveway, right to go right.

206 **How do I back up fast?**

When leaving your driveway, it's okay to turn around and look out the rear window so you can more easily check for traffic or pedestrians. But to drive backward with speed or for longer than a few feet, face forward and use your mirrors to see behind you. This gives you more contact with the steering wheel—crucially important, since the action of the wheel is magnified when in reverse—and puts you in your accustomed relationship with the accelerator and brake, preventing you from accidentally stepping on the wrong pedal.

207 What do I do to stop hydroplaning?

Do nothing. That queasy feeling that you're gliding on a large puddle or pool of water on the road is usually a momentary problem. Back off the gas without braking, and keep the wheel straight, despite the feeling of having lost contact with the road surface. That way, your tires will be headed in the right direction when you hit relatively dry road again.

208 What's the best way to drive in a blizzard?

Before you get on the road, start your car and turn on the front and rear defrosters. Then get out of the car and knock all the snow off the windows and hood so you are starting out with the best possible visibility. Make sure there's no ice built up on your windshield that will impede your wipers. Take a few minutes to plan your route to avoid hills if you can, since going up or down presents the most problems—for you and for others who might get in your way.

Once under way, stay to the middle of the road, where the crown of the road is flattest, and where you'll have the most space to make corrections if you begin to slide toward the shoulder or ditch. If it's safe, straddle the center of the road to keep yourself from sliding. Go slowly, braking only if you have to, and give the cars in front of you plenty of room.

209 **When should I downshift?**

Downshifting lets you gain speed more quickly or slow down with more control. A curving highway on-ramp, for instance, can often leave you overgeared, with little power. Downshift to restore your car's responsiveness to the accelerator. On the other hand, as you approach a stop, "engine-brake" by taking your foot off the accelerator and downshifting. (Remember that you'll be slowing without your brake lights giving warning to drivers behind you.) Downshifting, instead of braking, into a slowdown also means you'll be in the appropriate gear when it's time to speed up again.

210 **How do I speed without getting a ticket?**

Most police officers have in mind a certain range over the legal limit that they consider reasonable—from 9 to 15 mph. As the posted speed limit gets higher, however, these margins get smaller. Time of day matters, too: you're more likely to get stopped after 11 P.M., or in early morning or midafternoon, when school buses are on the road. At any speed, recklessness effects an officer's calculation—tailgating, weaving through traffic, or passing on the right can increase your chances of getting flagged down.

4
5
6

211 **How do I drive a motorcycle?**

It's a good idea to get the feel by riding on the back of a motorcycle before you handle it yourself. When it's your turn, start with the bike in neutral. (A green indicator will light up on the instrument panel.) Your main brakes and accelerator are in your right hand as you grip the handlebars. Your clutch is in your left hand, while the gearshift is at your left foot. Near your right foot is the rear-wheel brake.

Depress the clutch and kick down the shifter once to put it in first gear. As you let out the clutch very slowly, feel for the friction point. You don't need to add any gas at all at first. As you get comfortable with the friction point, you can roll the throttle back a small amount until you are properly under way and put your feet on the footrests. If you want to stop, pull in the clutch again and brake with your right hand, then with your right foot.

All the other gears are reached by kicking the shift up with the clutch in: once to get into second, again for third, up to fifth or sixth.

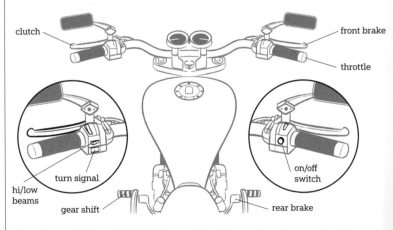

Some German, Italian, and British bikes may have the controls on the opposite side.

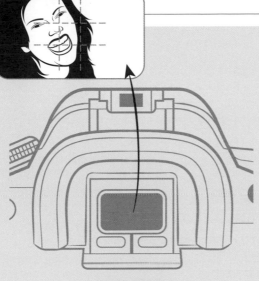

212 HOW DO I TAKE SOMEBODY'S PICTURE?

STEPHEN SHEFFIELD
photographer

"Keep things simple. Using a flash unnecessarily complicates things. If you can, use natural light. Don't use a tripod if you don't need to. Focusing your attention on the person is the first step in obtaining better people pictures.

"Use a wide aperture and a fast lens such as f2.8 to throw the background out of focus and to place emphasis on the subject. Even so, watch out for poles, trees, and bright colors, as they tend to stick out. Focus on the subject's eyes. If the eyes are out of focus, your whole picture will appear out of focus.

"Hold the camera vertically when photographing one person; horizontal for a group. Place your subject off center. Imagine a tic-tac-toe game on your camera's viewfinder. Place your subject where one of those lines intersect, and your composition will be more interesting than if you place the subject dead center."

1
2
3
4
5
6

GUYS' LIST ■

Ten songs every guy should have on his music player

1. **"RING OF FIRE"**
   Johnny Cash (1963)

2. **"(I CAN'T GET NO) SATISFACTION"**
   the Rolling Stones (1965)

3. **"TRY A LITTLE TENDERNESS"**
   Otis Redding (1966)

4. **"A DAY IN THE LIFE"**
   The Beatles (1967)

5. **"SEX MACHINE"**
   James Brown (1970)

6. **"THUNDER ROAD"**
   Bruce Springsteen (1975)

7. **"I WANNA BE SEDATED"**
   the Ramones (1978)

8. **"LONDON CALLING"**
   the Clash (1979)

9. **"LOSING MY RELIGION"**
   R.E.M. (1991)

10. **"SMELLS LIKE TEEN SPIRIT"**
    Nirvana (1991)

213 What do I need to drive across country?

Every guy should drive across the United States at least once. How you go depends on whether you're moving from one side of the country to the other, or just seeing the sights. Either way, here are a few things to consider to make the trip go smoothly:

▶ **SECURE A VEHICLE** If you already own a car, submit the tires, belts, and cooling system to a thorough inspection by a professional mechanic. Have him do any maintenance (like a timing-belt change or tune-up) that will come due on your trip.

No wheels? Renting makes economic sense only if you're making a beeline for the opposite coast. Car-transport companies engage drivers to deliver cars between distant cities, most often paying part or all of the gas—but again, you're given only a day or so over the minimum to make the trip.

▶ **PLOT YOUR COURSE** If you have a deadline, of course, you'll need to stick to the interstates. But if there's no need to rush, your drive should be a compilation of greatest hits: legendary stretches of road, punctuated by grand vistas and historic places (see page 102 for some tips). Whether it's your first time or your hundredth, you may want to organize your trip around a theme, like music, food, or national parks—tracking the blues from the Mississippi Delta to Chicago to New York, eating barbecue along the southern tier, or visiting every major public preserve from Yosemite to the Smoky Mountains. Plan your route down to where you'll stay each night, then be prepared to improvise, follow local advice, and simply meander.

▶ **HAVE A STRATEGY** A crew of drivers should agree on general parameters: two-hour driving shifts make for comfortable, alert drivers and are frequent enough to ward off constant pee stops, wheel hogs, or shirkers.

A strategy is more important for a solo crosser, for whom consistent breaks are more important. If sightseeing is not on the agenda, consider traveling at off-hours: on the road by 8 P.M., off the road as bars are about to close. Have a couple of stiff drinks and bed down until about noon. Lollygag as the suckers go about their workday, gumming up the roads. After dinner, gas up and head out again, disturbed neither by desert heat nor traffic jams.

214 **What should I bring on a major road trip?**

▶ **MUSIC** Whether you're burning rubber or wandering, music is an additional companion. Buy an adapter for your MP3 player to have your favorite tunes at your fingertips. Or—if you want to be old school—gather your core tunes on CDs. As any conurbation comes into view, tap into the local musical flavor by switching to your radio, which may alert you to some hot local concert or live-music joint. Specialty record stores are an excellent place to stretch your legs while replenishing your stock of tunes—if you go the CD route— snagging a rare piece of vinyl or finding out about the local music scene.

▶ **FOOD** Like music, snacks in the car keep you entertained and awake. Dry food—pretzels, chips, energy bars, and nuts—is easier to eat at 70 mph than messy sandwiches; it also keeps better. Mix in some fruit to keep your bodily functions on track despite your prolonged inactivity. A long road trip is a good time to develop bad habits, like gum chewing or drinking soda pop. If you don't entertain your taste buds, you'll tend to stop more frequently to distract yourself otherwise.

▶ **GADGETS** Pioneers in Conestoga wagons would have killed for a GPS route finder, which you can plug into your accessory charger. A mobile Internet hookup allows you to blog your trip and check alternate routes. A monitor for your car's onboard computer can plug in under your dashboard to diagnose engine ills.

MANLY ARTS

215 **What do I need to do to hail a cab in this city?**

In some places you call for a cab or get one at a designated taxi stand. But hailing a cab on the street should be second nature. Rain, rush hour, and fifteen minutes after a sporting event has ended are the toughest conditions in which to get a cab. It's a simple supply-and-demand problem, so your task is to improve your position against the competition. First, cabbies prefer customers who look like they are good for a decent tip. Tuck in your shirt, and take off any garments that give you a juvenile look—a hockey jersey, your backward-turned baseball hat. Now that you look suitable, position yourself at a corner where cabbies gliding by in two directions can see you. If traffic is going north, be on the south corner, and vice versa. Stick your arm unabashedly into the air and give your hand an occasional wave.

Taxis often indicate whether they are occupied, off duty, or available by means of a light on the roof.

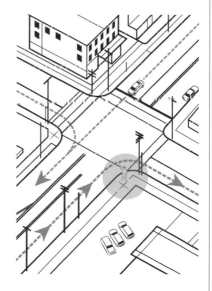

Positioning yourself at a corner is best.

Figure out the code so you don't wear yourself out yelling "Taxi!" at engaged cabs. In fact, don't yell; cabbies are good at spotting their fares. If you spot a cab unloading passengers ahead of you and don't think you're going to reach the door before it pulls away, give a loud whistle.

If the situation is desperate, don't try to beat out all comers. Approach another waver and ask if he wants to split the next cab. Or take off walking toward your destination, keeping an eye out for hotels where the cabbies are lined up for customers. Go inside the lobby for a minute, then exit and ask the doorman to get you a cab (tip him if he succeeds).

216 **How do I whistle loudly?**

Make a circle with your thumb and forefinger. Place the crease where your thumb and finger touch loosely against the tip of your tongue and inside your mouth slightly behind your teeth. Pull your lips in to

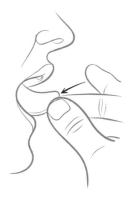

cover your teeth and clamp down firmly. Expel air out forcefully, adjusting the angle of your fingers against your tongue until you get a whistling sound.

Now that you can whistle, use the skill conservatively. Never whistle at a woman (except in private and in a low tone, as a compliment) or a grown person. But when calling dogs, passing ships, or cabbies, there's no reason to stint.

217 **How do I take good candids?**

When documenting a crowded event, take good pictures with abandon and sort them out later. Grab crowd shots by holding the camera above your head and clicking. Take portraits of people when they are unaware or too busy to pose. Don't tell someone to smile; tell him that he looks great or compliment her hair. Finding a rhythm in your shooting is more important than studied composition—it never fails that the shots you congratulated yourself for capturing will turn out to be blurred or stilted, while the random shot you got will be the gem.

218 **What's the best way to hold the camera steady?**

Your arms should form a triangle, with the camera clasped between your palms at the top point, and your elbows spread slightly and touching your sides so they are steadied against your ribs. Just before you take the picture, breathe in and lightly hold your breath. Push the button halfway to focus and click.

219 **Which camera should I buy?**

Assuming you're in the market for a digital camera, first consider how many megapixels you're looking for. Most reasonably priced digital cameras nowadays offer a resolution of at least five megapixels, plenty for the purposes of casual shooting. You only need more if you are intending to get artistic, and even then, seven is about the upper limit before you're seriously limiting the number of photos you can store on your computer's hard drive.

For recording holidays, birthdays, and the like, buy an inexpensive

1
2
3
4
5
6

point-and-shoot camera that will focus itself, choose the aperture and speed settings for you, and decide whether flash is necessary. You won't miss many candid shots with this kind of help.

A single-lens reflex camera is for you if you want to control depth of field, exposure, and flash. The viewfinder on these cameras will show precisely what will be recorded. They are also heavier, harder to operate, and more expensive.

220 **What's the best way to ice beer?**

"On" ice is a misnomer, since perching bottles and cans atop a pile of ice results in warm beer. Fill the beer box instead with an 80/20 mix of ice and water. Submerge the bottles up to their necks. Not only will the beer get cold sooner and stay cold longer, but the ice won't cut the hands of people rummaging for the beer they want.

If you're trying to chill beer quickly, give each bottle a quick spin (not a shake) every few minutes. This circulates the cooled liquid through the bottle.

221 **How do I tap a keg?**

Two things to consider well ahead of time: given the difficulty of coddling a 160-pound tank of beer, your keg has probably taken a few bumps on its way to the drinking site. So first, let the keg sit still, preferably in position and on ice, for as long as two hours before you tap it. And second, make sure you've got the right kind of tap: imported beer is tapped with a slightly different mechanism than domestic taps.

When the time comes to tap your keg, remove the plastic seal and line up the notches on the tap with the notches in the keg's opening. Push down hard, and without relenting turn the tap to the right until you can't turn it further. Push down on the handle and you're ready to pump. Pump as little as you need to get the beer flowing. No matter how gently you've treated your keg, and how cool it is, your first few pints are going to be foamy. Pour them and set them aside to resolve into beer before pouring your first guests' pints.

222 What can I use to open a beer without a bottle opener?

Several implements can be used when you're stranded without a beer opener. In each case, you may need to loosen the cap by degrees until you're practiced enough to get the cap off in one go.

▶ **PAPER** Make a three-quarter-inch fold at the bottom of a normal sheet of printer paper, then repeat until you've folded the entire paper. Now fold it once in the other direction. Ring the bottle's neck with your fingers less than an inch from the cap. Brace the paper's edge vertically between your forefinger and the cap's bottom rim and push up, using your finger as a fulcrum.

▶ **ANOTHER BEER** Tilt another bottle upside down and match the edge of each cap to the other. Pull up with consistent pressure until the first cap comes loose.

▶ **TEETH** Willing to risk chipping a tooth for a bottle of beer? Start by fitting your bottom row of teeth under the cap's edge

1
2
3
4
5
6

as your top row pinches down on the top of the cap. As soon as you hear the seal break, back off and finish the job with your hand.

EXPERT WITNESS

223 WHAT GAMES SHOULD I KNOW HOW TO PLAY?

CHRIS BAKER
games editor, *Wired* magazine

▶ **SUPER MARIO BROS.** "This is to games what *The Iliad* and *The Odyssey* are to literature. It's the archetypal game, and a lot of geek humor is centered around 'power-up mushrooms,' and other of the game's signifiers and icons."

▶ **MS. PAC-MAN GALAGA** "It pays to be well versed in at least one old-school arcade game, and this hybrid is one you'll find at a lot of bowling alleys and Laundromats."

▶ **GRAND THEFT AUTO** "Infamous as well as famous, it's another game whose terms, like asking someone their wanted level, have become taglines in the gamer world."

▶ **WORLD OF WARCRAFT** "The game is so highly addictive, it's like someone should know how to take a hit of crack. By this point it has been played by 12 million people, and has escaped the niche that most games exist in. It's sometimes referred to as nerd golf."

▶ **DUNGEONS & DRAGONS** "Not digital, but the old board game. We're sort of in a renaissance of Dungeons & Dragons these days, among older geeks who were into it as kids, but also younger players, because it's a badge of geek pride. The math of it is the cornerstone of every video game, the way certain attributes are quantified and health that can be diminished."

GAMES AND GAMBLING

224 **Which poker games do I need to know?**

Draw and stud poker used to dominate any friendly Friday-night game. But since poker became a televised sport, no-limit hold 'em, the most spectator-friendly form of poker, has become king. Here are some games you should know.

▶ **TEXAS HOLD'EM** The most popular game these days, Texas Hold'em is also one of the easiest to grasp. Working with two "hole" cards of your own and five communal cards placed faceup in the middle of the table, you fashion your best hand while deducing what others may have.

Play starts when each of the two players sitting to the dealer's left bets a small, predetermined amount of money or chips to seed the pot, called "little blind" and the "big blind." The dealer then flips two cards to each player, facedown. On the strength of those cards, each player bets. Three cards are dealt showing to the center of the table, with bets being placed after the third. A fourth and fifth card follow, with bets on each. When all the players are finished betting, the hands are revealed.

▶ **OMAHA** Omaha is hold'em played with four hole cards instead of two, resulting in better hands all around and more action. Your hand is still composed of two hole cards and three communal cards. Omaha hi-lo is played identically as hold'em, but the low hand splits the pot with the high hand. If you can make both high and low hands with the same seven cards, you swipe the whole pot. If you're playing with an eight-or-better rule, a low hand with a card over eight is disqualified from the pot and the high hand takes it all.

▶ **STUD** Similar to hold'em, but for many traditionalists' money, a grittier, more suspenseful game. Each player gets two cards down and one up. Bets ensue, starting with low card showing. Then each player gets three more cards of his or her own, faceup, with a bet placed after each, this time led by the player with the best hand showing. The final card is placed facedown, and after a final round of betting, hands are revealed.

▶ **RAZZ** Razz is a race for the bottom. The dealing imitates stud, but the worst-possible hand takes the pot, with all straights and flushes discounted and aces low. The "best" hand in razz is the ace through five cards. Second "best" is ace through four with a six.

▶ **HORSE** A round-robin of hold'em, Omaha, razz, stud, and eight-or-better hi-lo stud played in succession, changing each time the deal passes to the next player.

▶ **DRAW** After an ante, each player is dealt five cards, and bets on their initial hand. Players can exchange up to three of their cards in the hope of bettering their hand (four cards under some rules if the player is holding an ace). Another round of betting precedes the reveal.

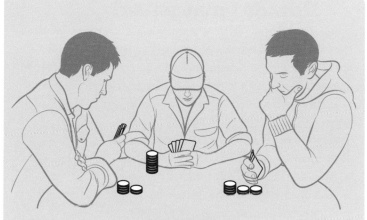

EXPERT WITNESS

225 HOW DO I KEEP A POKER FACE?

ALEX OUTHRED
professional poker player and founder, DeepStacksUniversity.com

"The term 'poker face' isn't really broad enough. It's your whole poker demeanor. Keep your behavior simple. Watch out for nervous tics or any pacifying motions like rubbing your arms or your face. If you can't control it, cover it up: I found that I would bite my lip, so now I rest my face on my hand and cover my mouth. The best way to control your movements is to develop routines, like a basketball player does at a free throw line or a batter at the plate. They help you relax, so whether things are good or bad you can be—or at least look—consistent."

226 **How do I play poker?**

Once you know the hierarchy of poker hands, you can get the hang of any variation on the game. At a friendly gathering, most guys are happy to show you the ropes of their favorite variation, but never go to a poker table without knowing what beats what. From lowest to highest, here are the potentially winning hands:

- ▶ **Pair** Any two cards of the same value, or rank.
- ▶ **Two pair** Any four cards made up of pairs.
- ▶ **Three of a kind** Any three cards of the same rank.
- ▶ **Straight** Five cards of consecutive values. Aces can have the value of one (low), or can top a king (high).
- ▶ **Flush** Five cards of the same suit.
- ▶ **Full house** Three cards of one rank, with two cards of another.
- ▶ **Four of a kind** Four cards, all of the same rank.
- ▶ **Straight flush** Five cards of the same suit of consecutive rank.
- ▶ **Royal straight flush** Ace, king, queen, jack, ten of the same suit.

In the case of similar hands, the hand made of cards of higher value wins. A pair of queens beats a pair of fives, for example, and a royal flush beats one with no face cards.

227 **What are the rules of card-table etiquette?**

Your buds normally glory in rude noises and loutish behavior, but a card table calls everyone to a higher standard. Horseplay distracts from play and tests losers' sore tempers. There's too much objection-able behavior to list, but to get an idea, check out Paul Newman's

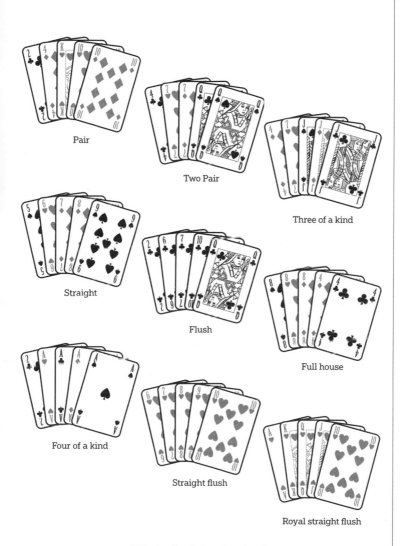

Pair

Two Pair

Three of a kind

Straight

Flush

Full house

Four of a kind

Straight flush

Royal straight flush

Winning hands in order of rank

drunken burping, swearing, spilling turn at the poker table on a train in the 1973 movie *The Sting*.

More hard-and-fast are the rules about handling and viewing the cards.

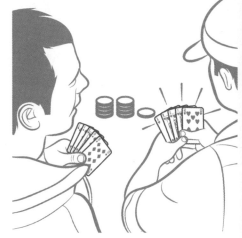

▶ Don't let cards fall to the floor or go below the tabletop, where they could theoretically be exchanged for others.

▶ Don't touch anyone else's cards or the communal cards. It's customary not to look at your cards before everyone has received theirs.

▶ Don't touch anyone else except in the most casual game.

▶ Refrain from commenting on others' play or in general jabbering too much or being a nuisance. If you're not playing a hand, observe from a place where you can't see anyone's cards, and at all costs don't kibitz, or help any player make his or her decisions.

228 **How do I bluff?**

There are two ways to win a hand. One is to have the best cards, which amounts to luck. The other way is to get your opponents to fold by playing aggressively, betting forcefully but intelligently, even when the cards aren't there. Like any strategy, bluffing is best implemented when the odds and the situation complement your attack.

You'll be more convincing if you bluff when you're positioned far from the dealer, when your bets are coming after everyone or almost everyone has already placed theirs. Step up the bet slowly, so you don't blow the other players out of the hand before they have a chance to give up their chips. Pace yourself by making your moves in reaction to the progress of the deal, reinforcing the idea that you were looking for a card and got it. By that time, too, you'll likely have fewer opponents in the hand: it's easier to bluff one guy off his iffy bet if it's just you and him left.

Pay attention to what has been dealt and try to form a good idea of what the competition is holding: you can't represent a hand your opponent already has.

Lastly, bluff rarely. Each time your hand doesn't back up your bravado, you lose credibility. Take a page from Clooney in *Ocean's Eleven*, and get bluffy when you're holding an unbeatable hand. The idea is to keep the table off balance, not for one hand, but for the entire night.

229 **When should I bet?**

Each variation of poker has its particular schedule of dealing and betting. In general, you have to make a decision about betting whenever you receive more information about the quality of your hand. When deciding what to bet, consider the odds that you have a winning hand.

You can find the odds of winning with various hands in poker manuals and online. Hint: memorize the bottom of the chart—the odds of winning with relatively common pairs and three of a kind. When you're holding a hand with decent odds, you can bet confidently but not extravagantly. When you have an excellent hand, don't blow everyone out of the water with your betting early. Nurse your opponents along in order to encourage them to bet before you spring your trap.

230 **When do I go all-in?**

"All-in" has entered the cultural lexicon, where it means pulling off the ultimate power play. Ironically, one of the best times to go all-in is when you're not in a position of power at all: when your chip pile has dwindled to the point that you're going to have trouble making it through the next few rounds of betting. You may have your back against the wall, but giving yourself only one way out will look like confidence to your opponents. Even when you're desperate, make sure your bet matches the odds: your return on your bet should reflect your hand's likelihood of winning.

231 **How do I keep the betting from getting out of hand?**

Agree to a pot limit or a spread limit. In pot-limit games, players may raise only the value of the pot. A spread limit sets a low end of the spread—usually the ante, say a nickel or a dollar, and an upper end of the spread, a quarter or five dollars. At no time can any player bet or raise less than the lower figure or more than the higher one.

232 **How do I play online poker?**

Playing poker on the Internet is illegal, citizen. The poker sites that meet with U.S. government approval are the ".net" versions that merely educate you to better play their offshore sister sites where real money is wagered. Got that?

For those who venture onto those offshore sites, which require you to download their software to play, the rules are no different, but the texture of the game changes profoundly. With no physical cards to shuffle and deal and no body language to read, speed becomes the defining force—a hundred hands can be played in the time it takes to play fifty at a live table. This frenetic pace is heightened by players who participate in several games at once. In this environment, quick mathematical calculation and hand recognition is everything. Some players contend that virtual tells are discernible to experienced players, but as a beginner, your best bet is to keep your odds and "outs" charts handy.

233 **What are the rules of blackjack?**

Beginners in Vegas gravitate toward blackjack because there are relatively few variables—the winning hand is simple to recognize and your only opponent is the dealer. The goal is to gather a hand as close to twenty-one in value as you can get without going over. (Face cards are worth ten and aces can be counted as a one or an eleven.) There is an initial bet, the dealer gives you a card facedown and one faceup, and you can either ask for more cards or stand. (In multideck casino games, both cards are dealt faceup.) The dealer's hand must take more cards until his or her hand totals at least seventeen.

Sound simple? Depend on gamblers and casinos to complicate even the most straightforward betting game. If you are dealt two cards of the same value, you can split your hand into two and play them consecutively. You can double your bet after you get your first two cards (often incurring some restrictions on how many additional cards you can take). You can choose to surrender halfway through a hand and forfeit only half your bet.

234 How do I count cards?

The team of MIT students featured in the book *Bringing Down the House* made card counting look like an exotic and dangerous game for people with calculators in their heads. In reality, card counting can be a pretty simple method of expanding on the casino's already fairly crappy odds at the blackjack table.

The basic principle is that the house, which has to take cards until it makes seventeen, prefers to have lower-value cards in the pipeline, while players prefer face cards that will get them quickly to twenty (forcing the dealer to beat them with twenty-one). To keep track of how many face cards and lower-value cards have been dealt from the present deck, start on an imaginary number line at zero. When you see any card worth less than seven, add one point. When you see any card worth ten or more, subtract a point. (Seven, eight, and nine are neutral and worth zero.) The higher the count, the more you bet.

235 **What are the rules of roulette?**

Your first move is to sit down at the table. Anyone sitting at the table is considered in—don't be the onlooking chump who sits down and doesn't intend to play. As soon as the bets for the previous round are finished being paid out, place your betting chip (roulette often has two sets: one for placing bets, one for cashing out) on a square that represents your wager. After the dealer, or croupier, has launched the ball on the spinning wheel, he will announce the end of betting. When you've won, the dealer will usually deposit your winnings on the square you've just won with. Keep your eyes on your fries or you'll end up duplicating your previous bet.

The most straightforward bet is made by placing a chip directly on a number. You can also make other inside bets—those placed on the number grid—by placing your chips on the line dividing two numbers (a split), on the corner of four number squares (a corner), on the outside line on either end of a row of numbers (street bet) or two rows (double street), or the corner of a row and either the zero

00	3	6	9	12	15	18	21	24	27	30	33	36	2 to 1
	2	5	8	11	14	17	20	23	26	29	32	35	2 to 1
0	1	4	7	10	13	16	19	22	25	28	31	34	2 to 1
	1st 12				2nd 12				3rd 12				
	1to18		EVEN		RED		BLACK		ODD		19 to 36		

1
2
3
4
5
6

or double-zero square (five-number). The single number bet pays its odds: 35–1. The payout on the multiple numbers decreases as you add winning squares.

Outside bets refer to those placed outside the number grid. Most are self-explanatory: a chip on the red or black square wins any bet of the same color; 1–18 wins when any number in the range comes up. (The squares marked "2–1" are the exception, paying those odds when any number in their rank comes up.)

236 **How do I play craps?**

If roulette plays the way it looks, craps is a thicket of arcane bets and twisty drama. The basic action is to bet for or against the probability that a dice roll will add up to seven: a three and a four, five and two,

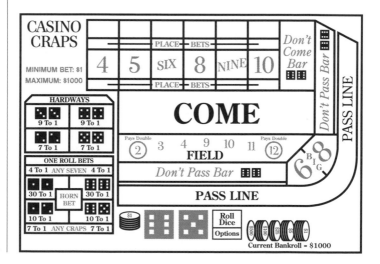

one and six. Want to bet that the shooter will roll seven on the first roll? Put your chips on the "Pass Line." Want to bet the opposite? Play "Don't Pass."

If the first roll comes to any number between four and ten, the total on the dice—called the point—is recorded by a white "puck" on a number chart. The shooter rolls again. If the point turns up again before seven does, Pass Line bets pay; Don't Pass loses. If the shooter rolls Craps—two, three, or twelve—before rolling a seven, Pass Line loses, and Don't Pass wins. Whenever a shooter wins or loses, the dice pass to the next player in clockwise order.

The rest of the bets on the craps board are side bets, on whether the shooter will make the point the "hard way"—by rolling doubles, or whether a six, eight, or both will come before seven, or on single-roll totals. Your safest bets are your Pass Line and Don't Pass, and it's best to stick to these until you're comfortable with the customs of the craps table—the most important of which apply to how you roll the dice: don't blow on them, talk about anyone needing new shoes, or toss so the dice fly off the table

237 **What's the procedure for betting on a horse?**

The betting window at the racetrack can be daunting for a beginner, so the first rule is to have your mind made up and your rap down. When you reach the window, place your bet in this order:

- ▶ Name of the track where your horse is running (most tracks allow you to bet on out-of-town races as well as theirs)
- ▶ The number of the race you are betting on

▶ The amount you are betting

▶ The type of bet you are making (win, place, or show)

▶ Identify the horse or horses you are wagering on by number, not by name

Example: "At Belmont Park, 5th race: $10 to win on the 7."

238 **How do I pick a winning horse?**

Take a look at any bettor at the track. What's he got that you don't? No, not the bad plaid jacket or the cigarette tucked behind his ear. It's *The Daily Racing Form.* Available at many a newspaper kiosk, the *DRF,* as it's known, lists the past performances of each horse running in your area. (The *DRF* is national, but is printed in regional editions.) Each horizontal line describes a horse's last dozen races—the quality of its competition, its position in the pack during the race, even how it ran (e.g., that it was doing fine until it was bumped hard by another horse). This wealth of data amounts to far too much information for a newbie to consider. But a few signals can help you get a handle on which horse has legs.

▶ **ODD HORSE OUT** Find the figure that tells you where the horse was positioned during the running of its races. Those horses that spent most of the race in the one or two spot running on or very near the lead are front-runners who tend to spend their energy too early. A horse with a higher number—a five or six—is learning how to hang back and make its move when the front-runners are spent. Even if it hasn't won yet, the next race may be the charm.

▶ **THE CLASS DROP** At the track, the best horses run in stakes races, those of middling quality are in "allowance" races; at the lower end are "claiming" races. When a horse thought good enough for stakes races has been losing consistently and is downgraded, its first races in a lower class present an opportunity.

▶ **THE SPRING BLOSSOM** A key tool in the *DRF* is a bold-faced number called the Beyer Speed Figure—never mind for now the intricacies of the Beyer figure's statistical provenance, but some horse-racing analysts have noted that when a three-year-old horse (like the colts and fillies that run the Triple Crown races) matches his best Beyer number recorded in his two-year-old year, a large jump in performance follows five or six weeks later. This pattern has been borne out in twenty of the past thirty Triple Crown races, leading canny bettors to such winners as Lemon Drop Kid (29–1) and Birdstone (35–1) in the Belmont Stakes.

239 **How do I play pool?**

Most pool is played sociably, meaning as something to do while drinking beer. You don't have to be tremendously skilled to hit the mark in these situations, but you don't want your lack of game to ruin a night out either.

Pick a straight cue—it shouldn't wobble when you roll it on the pool table's surface—with a decent tip. Rub the tip lightly on the edge, not the deep divot, of the cube of chalk.

Line up your shot while standing behind the numbered ball. Visualize the point on the ball your cue stick would have to hit to tap it directly into the pocket. Return to your place behind the cue, keeping an eye on that spot, and focus on it as you bend to take your shot. Find a comfortable position with your head in line with and overlooking your shot. Hold the cue firmly at the fatter end, with the point end resting on your thumb and held in place with your forefinger.

240 **Which ball do I hit?**

The most common game in pool halls is eight ball, in which the object is to knock in either all the striped balls or all the solid balls before knocking in the eight as the coup de grâce. You can also lose the game by sinking the eight before all your balls are off the table, or by scratching after pocketing the eight.

Strictly, the choice of stripes or solids is made by the first player to sink a ball after the break—a ball that goes in on the break decides nothing. In most pool halls, you'll find the rules are more lax, and the choice will be established if a ball drops on the break.

Strictly, too, each eight-ball shot must contact both an object ball and a rail (the formal name of a side bumper) or you give up your turn and your opponent gets the cue ball in hand to place it anywhere on the table. The Billiard Congress of America also stipulates that any shot whose object ball and intended pocket is not obvious must be called. In many casual games, however, rails normally don't come into play and calling is not enforced, except when shooting for the eight. The turn changes when either player fails to hole a ball.

All combination shots—using a colored ball in combination with the cue to strike and sink the object ball—are legal except one using the eight. (Local rules, however, often demand that you may only combo your own balls.)

Scratches—shots that sink the cue ball and balls jumped off the table—turn the cue ball over to your opponent to place anywhere on the table. Balls pocketed on scratches remain pocketed and jumped balls are not replaced. Scratching on the eight ball loses you the game. For complete rules, go to www.pool-table-rules.com.

241 **What can I do to sink a shot like a hustler?**

People expect you to make the head-on pool shot, even though it can be one of the toughest shots for a beginner. Instead, look for a ball loitering around a side pocket. Standing with the ball in question between you and the pocket, picture the spot where you'd hit the object ball directly with your cue stick to tap it in. Keep your eye on the spot as you walk

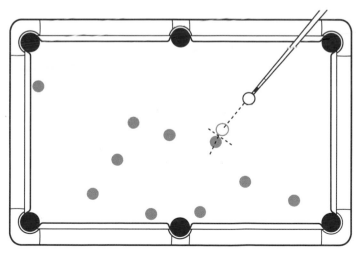

Aim the tip of your cue at the center of the cue ball.

back to the cue ball and line up your shot. You want the cue ball to barely glance the spot with its extreme edge, with just enough oomph to reach the pocket. Rolling in a slow kiss shot looks authoritative, and will inspire more aahs than jamming a ball into the corner.

242 How do I put English on the ball?

Anyone can make a fancy pool shot. What separates the men from the boys is being able to leave yourself a makable following shot. The underlying technique is called putting English, or spin, on the cue ball so that it ends up where you want it. To make a ball stop when it hits the object ball, tilt your stick downward as you strike the cue, so that the point of impact is very low on the ball. This causes the cue ball first to shoot forward, slide, and then stop when it hits the object ball.

Sometimes you want the cue ball to rebound off a rail (side cushion surrounding the playing surface) and cross the table to your next shot. You can control this rebound by spinning the cue right or left as you strike. If you want the cue ball to stay to the left of its natural rebound, strike it just left of center as you shoot. To keep it right, hit it right of center. After lots of practice, you'll be able to predict the path of the rebounding cue ball accurately.

Note: don't put English on the cue ball when you break or it will likely leave the table.

243 How do I play darts?

A dartboard is divided into an array of pie-slice shapes from one to twenty. Landing a dart in the black or yellow (or white) divisions of

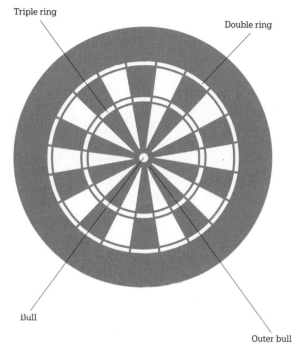

Triple ring

Double ring

Bull

Outer bull

those shapes earns you the points as numbered. Landing one in the outer narrow ring (often green and red) doubles your points; the inner ring triples them. Hitting the outside circle of the bull's-eye is worth twenty-five points, and the inner circle fifty. Each player gets three darts and tosses them all in each turn.

Traditionally, darts are played downward: you get a given number of points—again, tradition dictates 501 (or any three-digit number ending in 01)—and the point total of each turn is subtracted (usually on a nearby chalkboard) from your starting number. If you subtract past zero, or fail to zero out with a double, that turn is forfeited and the game continues.

244 **What are the rules of liar's dice?**

It used to be that a manly type of pub would have a few leather cups containing five or so dice sitting around. If you spot a dice setup today, you know you're in the right type of place. One use for these dice is to play draw poker, with pairs, two pairs, three of a kind, straights, full houses, and four of a kind the only possible hands.

Another dice-and-cup diversion is liar's dice, in which each player shakes a cup of five dice and then turns his cup over on the playing surface so his dice are trapped inside. He peeks at his dice and based on the numbers showing on his dice estimates how many of the same number are held by all the players. For instance, if he has two twos in his cup, he can bid four twos, wagering that his fellows are harboring at least two more twos. The player to his left can raise the bid by estimating a higher occurrence of twos, or make his own bid using a higher dice number. Or he can challenge the previous player's bid.

A round is ended when every player challenges the active bid. If the bid proves correct, the challengers sacrifice one of their dice. If the bid fails, the bidder loses a die. Play then continues until one die is left; its owner wins.

The game has also been played using the serial numbers on dollar bills. When a bidder wins, he extracts a dollar from each challenger.

BUFFING UP

245 **How do I get a workout with dumbbells?**

Maybe it's the name, but dumbbells are underrated. You can get a complete workout with dumbbells and an exercise ball. Push yourself to add weight as you get stronger, and incorporate different exercises into your routine. Try these:

▶ To work your **shoulders**, sit on an exercise ball with your feet flat on the floor, a dumbbell in each hand held above your shoulders, so your arms form an L shape and the dumbbells are about even with your ears [a]. Fully extend one arm [b] then the other [c], alternating until you can't raise the weight without breaking form. Take a break and do another set. Start with ten pounds on each side and work your way up.

▶ For **tricep** building, lie on your inflatable ball with the ball between your shoulder blades and your feet on the ground. Hold a dumbbell in each hand with your arms extended toward the ceiling [a]. Slowly bend your arms so the dumbbell passes your ear [b]. Pause, and raise the dumbbell to full extension again. This is harder than it sounds; start with light weights and build up.

▶ Lying on the ball again, hold a dumbbell in each hand with your arms extended away from your body, elbows slightly bent [a]. To work your **chest**, lift the dumbbells so they meet above your chest [b] and then back outward [c]. Repeat until you have a difficult time extending your arms.

4

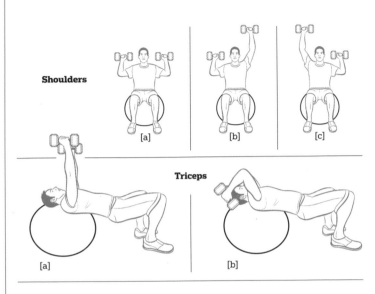

Shoulders

[a]　[b]　[c]

Triceps

[a]　[b]

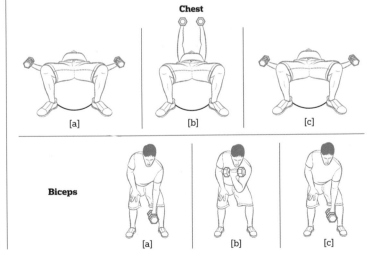

Chest

[a]　[b]　[c]

Biceps

[a]　[b]　[c]

▶ To get buff **biceps**, stand with your feet shoulder-width apart with a dumbbell in one hand. Lean forward, bending your knees but keeping your back straight until your arm hangs straight down. Rest your empty hand palm down on the near-side thigh [a]. Curl the dumbbell upward until it's almost touching your face [b], then slowly let it back down [c]. Repeat until you can't keep form, then switch hands.

246 **How do I bench-press my weight?**

For reasons that are unclear, gym lore has it that a guy should be able to bench-press his own weight. Here's how to build up to your weight in iron.

Lie back on a weight bench. With your feet on the ground (when trying to reach maximum weight, you need your feet to be stable so you can throw every muscle into the mix), lift a moderate weight for three repetitions. Increase the weight and do three more reps. Work your way up until you can't lift the weight more than once. Then decrease the weight in the same increments as you built up, using three repetitions each time.

Lift every other day, and at each session try to push your top weight, even by the smallest increments. It's important that you progress, but slowly. Expect to lift at least five weeks before you are able to lift your weight.

1
2
3
4
5
6

247 **How do I get a ripped chest?**

Regular push-ups will give your chest all the bulk and definition you need. Lying facedown with your toes perpendicular to the floor, position your hands so they are directly below your shoulders. Push your entire body off the floor with your hands until your arms are extended. Repeat as long as you can keep your back flat.

As you increase your repetitions, play with the position of your arms by moving them wide and out to the sides, or narrow with your thumbs touching, even forward or back to change which segment of your pecs (and triceps) is getting worked.

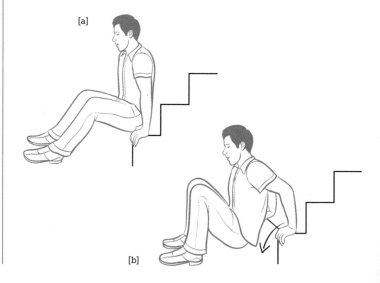

[a]

[b]

248 **What are easy exercises to do anywhere?**

There are ways to get fit without any weights or exercise paraphernalia, so you can work out without hitting the gym.

Try this one to work your **triceps**. Sit on the lowest step of a staircase and place your hands on the step above and behind you. Lift your backside by extending your arms [a]. Move forward and down toward the floor, and back up to sitting [b]. Repeat as many times as you can. The position of your feet will determine how difficult this exercise is: moving your feet away from your body makes it harder.

To work your **back,** lie down on the floor like Superman flying: arms out, forehead touching the floor [c]. Pick up your head and upper body at same time and see how long you can hold the position [d]. The trick is to keep your head in the same position as you started so you don't stretch the neck.

If your **legs** need toning, face a wall, standing with your fingers on the wall for balance; the lighter the touch, the better. Rise up on your toes as high as you can, slowly up and slowly down. As this exercise gets easier, let go of the wall.

[c]

[d]

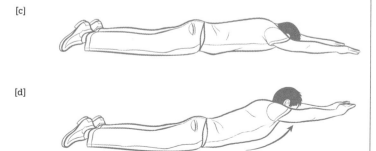

249 **How do I get the kind of abs the French girls call a "chocolate bar"?**

Developed abs may improve your love life, but they do a lot more than that: strong stomach muscles cause you to move more smoothly when walking or playing ball, give you better balance, and in the long run will help prevent lower back pain.

Here's a good exercise to get that six-pack. Lie on your back, knees bent, feet on the floor [a]. Interlace your fingers behind your head where the base of your skull meets your neck. Pull your shoulders up and forward, without pulling on your head with your arms. Lift yourself no higher than it takes to clear shoulder blades from the floor. Rotate your trunk as you come up by directing your left elbow toward the right knee, then alternate as you repeat [b]. Do as many as you can as long as you can maintain good form.

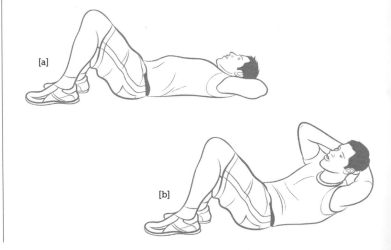

[a]

[b]

Killer moves

The four exercises below strengthen your major muscle groups, sharpen your mental focus, improve balance, and make severe demands on your cardio-pulmonary system, all while keeping you out of the weight room. Which is to say they are all guts and no glory. Are you man enough?

CROSS-COUNTRY SKIING During those winter months when you're otherwise sedentary, this is your chance to sweat in zero-degree weather.

SWIMMING WITH HAND PADDLES This all-over muscle builder raises swimming's otherwise low injury rate because it jacks up the load of the workout and puts extra stress on your shoulders. That means you have to be a little more careful, but you'll notice quickly the difference from regular swimming.

TAI CHI CHUAN This martial-art form is more akin to performing ballet in super-slo-mo than fighting. But it gives away nothing for building core strength, agility, and balance, and the intense focus required leaves your brain tingling.

VINYASA YOGA Not just for the ladies, this vigorous yoga practice will work all your major muscle groups, increase your flexibility, sharpen your mental focus, and give you a killer cardio sweat.

1
2
3
4
5
6

Guys' grub

The perfect foods for sports events, drinking nights, and other simple celebrations.

CHILI This everything-but-the-kitchen-sink dish appeals to a guy's tendency to cook by agglomeration. To a guileless can of tomatoes, add a can or two of beans, chili powder, a bay leaf, water, and a cup of beer; improvise with beef, pork or sausage, vegetables, and different bean varieties.

BARBECUE A guy can make a hobby of sampling hickory-smoked pork and other meats in all their regional varieties, seeking out smoky shacks down country lanes or the storefronts that have a line out the door on Friday nights. Appoint yourself a connoisseur and you'll have a way to connect with locals wherever you go.

RAW OYSTERS The prospect of downing a half-dozen creatures with the consistency of snot may seem more like a hazing rite than an appetizer. But after you acquire the taste—aided by an icy brew and judicious seasoning with hot sauce, horseradish, or cocktail sauce—you'll find yourself yearning for their refreshingly briny sting.

PIZZA If you grew up on the national chains, you'll always have an abiding affection for breadlike crust and flavorless sauce. But nowadays many towns have sprouted a pie shop with a wood-fired oven and an ambitious beer menu. It's a model that promises a golden age for hungry guys.

250 **How do I do a flip turn?**

The flip turn is what transforms swimming from a recreational activity into a workout. Begin thinking about the turn about five feet out while swimming full speed. It takes practice to get the distance right:

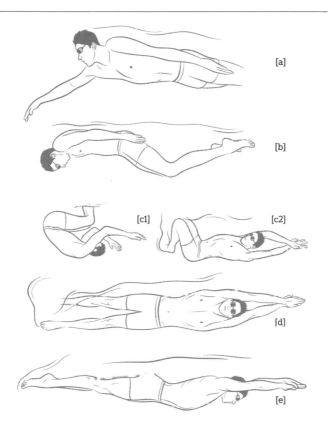

[a]

[b]

[c1] [c2]

[d]

[e]

you want to be close enough that you have momentum to carry you toward the wall, but far enough that you have time to flip [a]. Forcefully tuck your head down and slightly to one side and pull your body into a crouch [b]. Cup your hands and bring them up as if you were tossing something over your shoulders [c1]. This motion will cause your feet to flip over [c2]. Twist so that you are close to right side up when your feet hit the wall [d]. The timing should be such that your legs are bent as your feet contact the wall so you can quickly extend the knees to propel yourself off of the wall [e].

EATING OUT/EATING IN

251 **How do I tell a good restaurant from a mediocre one?**

You can tell a lot by analyzing the menu. A good restaurant concentrates on a few things, with one to three entrées in each category. A menu with a voluminous list of dishes—say, seven chicken, five veal, and six fish—probably doesn't do any one of them well. But getting a good meal is also a matter of how you order.

Never ask, "What's good here?" Ask what the chef is excited about, or what he's particularly proud of. If you order what the chef is psyched to cook that night, you may get some extras added to your meal. The chef may even visit your table to ask if you enjoyed it, which always impresses a date.

252 **What can I do to get into a "hot" restaurant?**

Even when the newest hot spot in town is all booked up for months in advance, you know they could make a table appear if Brad Pitt arrived. But slipping the maître d' a twenty doesn't make you Brad Pitt. When a restaurant is new, the only hope you have is to work a connection—does your uncle's accountant also do the books for the place?—or to show up at an odd hour, say for the 10 P.M. seating, and hope for the best. Dress appropriately, be polite, and stress your interest in the restaurant, not the paparazzi scene. ("We love great food. Is there anything you can do for us?" is a nice place to start.) If there's a cancellation, the reservations agent might take pity on you.

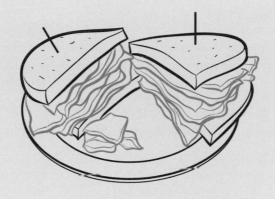

253 HOW DO I ORDER A CLASSIC DELI SANDWICH?

SANFORD LEVINE
owner, Carnegie Deli, Manhattan

"In a deli, rye bread is the bread that's recommended. Rye is synonymous with delis. If you come in here and you ask for white bread, we look at you as if you had horns. You only use mustard—we have a German mustard that's made to our own formulas and you put it on pastrami and corned beef. We get people from all over. Sometimes they come in and ask for tuna fish. We say, 'You traveled three thousand miles to eat tuna fish?' That's it. Meat and mustard on rye bread. Some old-timers who were born and raised in New York put coleslaw on, too, which is acceptable. We've been open seventy-two years. If it ain't broke, we ain't fixing it."

Tables at more established places can be a tough get for Saturday-night dinner, less so for lunch or a weeknight meal. Frequenting an eatery when business is slow, and chatting up the staff when they have a moment to breathe, may pay off when you want to take some out-of-town friends for dinner during prime time.

254 Should I order wine by the glass or bottle?

Wine by the glass is a better deal if you and your dinner companion are really having just one. But restaurants count on you to order a second, at which point they collect. (See page 225 for tips on picking the right kind.) When in doubt, go for the bottle. In many states it's now legal to cork a wine bottle you haven't finished and take it home.

255 Can I bring my own bottle to a restaurant?

If it's BYOB, no problem—that's the only way you'll get wine with dinner because the restaurant doesn't have a liquor license so it

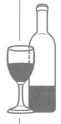

can't sell you any wine. Otherwise, it depends on the corkage fee—the charge the restaurant adds to the bill for serving your bottle. Corkage fees can run to fifty or a hundred dollars in some establishments while even rather sophisticated ones can charge as little as ten dollars. If your wine sets you back twenty dollars in a store, you'll pay forty to fifty for the same wine in a restaurant. So call ahead and calculate your savings.

256 What's the proper way to order wine?

The worst move you can make, in a restaurant or beyond, is to pretend to have knowledge you don't. By all means browse the wine list for a specific wine you recognize (and like), but if you don't know a vintner from a vintage, don't try to fake it. The same goes for the kabuki of approving a wine you've ordered. Forgo the swirling and smelling— unless you really know what you're looking for, you're just making an ass of yourself. If the waiter pours you a small amount to sample, take a sip. Unless the stuff is vinegar, nod affirmatively and get on with your meal.

That's not to say you can't apply a few easy-to-remember parameters to make sense of the wine list:

▶ **PAIR FLAVORS, NOT COLORS** The dictum about drinking red wine with meat and white with fish is at best imprecise. Your choice of wine should be determined by what's on the menu. Match Thai food with a white that cuts through its spicy heat: a crisp sauvignon blanc or a fruity Gewürtztraminer. Deep reds go with steak, yes, but they also complement anything with tomato sauce.

▶ **STAY UNDER TWENTY-FIVE DOLLARS** Your father's mistake was spending too little; yours might be spending too much. Spend more than fifty dollars or less than a hundred and you're likely getting neither a great deal nor a great wine. A domestic wine for fifteen to twenty-five dollars is apt to get you both.

▶ **PACIFIC WAVE** The best deals and most crowd-pleasing wines these days come from the New World: California and Chile have been producing excellent, affordable reds. The most surprising whites lately hail from the other side of the Pacific, from New Zealand, while Australian reds have become dependably interesting.

If all else fails, ask your waiter to recommend something, or ask him to send over the sommelier. They may try to steer you toward a pricey bottle, in which case you're within your rights to ask for something a little more reasonable or, if your date's looking on, bite your lip and scan the list further until you've come across something in your price range.

EXPERT WITNESS

257 WHY DO WE MARINATE MEAT?

STEVEN RAICHLEN
author of *Planet Barbecue!* and host of *The Primal Grill* on PBS

"A marinade is like the makeup a beautiful woman might apply. It enables you to give food an enhanced identity. You can introduce ethnic influences, say a Mexican flavor with cilantro and tequila, Italian with oregano, Thai with lemongrass, or South African with piri-piri chilies. The other primary use of marinades is to keep, say, your food from drying out on the grill. Most are not difficult to put together, but you have to leave time for them to penetrate—from fifteen minutes with shrimp and other fish to four hours for a standard steak to overnight for a cut of meat like a pork shoulder."

258 **Should I buy a charcoal or gas grill?**

The big question is which kind to get—charcoal or gas? Gas grills are more expensive and take up more space, but fire up more quickly and there's less of a mess than with a charcoal grill. Charcoal, however, lends food a more authentic, smoky taste, and allows you to experiment with wood, flavored briquettes, and other fuel—not to mention the pure caveman pleasure of starting your own fire.

259 **How do I start a charcoal grill?**

Begin with a device called a chimney starter, which looks like a tin milk pitcher without a bottom. (Square ones, rarer but increasingly available, are better.) Place the chimney on the grill grate, stuff the

bottom third with newspaper, and fill to the top with your charcoal. No lighter fluid needed: light the newspaper and in about fifteen minutes your coals will be uniformly glowing orange and ready to spread on the grate.

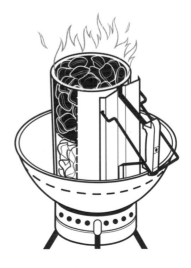

Prefer pyrotechnics? Mound your charcoal at the center of the grate and douse it liberally with lighter fluid. Allow the fluid a minute or so to soak into the briquettes, then light several briquettes at their edges until the fire catches. You've done your job when you have a roaring fire independent of the lighter fluid's initial flare-up. As soon as the white coals glow orange when you blow on them, distribute them for cooking.

260 What's the best way to grill the perfect burger?

The prep for a perfectly grilled burger is the same whatever your heat source: roll hamburger meat gently into a ball, squish flat (for rare), flatter (medium), or flattest (well done), salt and pepper both sides, and put it on the grill.

The difference lies in your choices before and after the grill. Over the unmediated heat of a live flame, the meat tends to dry out, so pick beef that's a little fattier than you'd want for pan-fried burgers: 85 percent lean will do. When the burgers barely give when you poke them, direct them immediately to a toasted bun covered with a leaf of lettuce to keep the juices from being absorbed by the bun. Grilling guru Steve Raichlen (see Expert Witness, page 226) suggests juicing the burger's fat content by hiding a bit of butter inside the patty, and buttering the bun after you toast it.

261 How do I grill fish?

Fish can be slippery devils, and it's no different on the grill. Fillets, especially, break apart as you try to flip, move, or remove them. Any thin piece of fish should be clamped inside a fish basket, a device that looks like two toddler snowshoes clapped together. In a pinch you can wrap the fish in foil, but you'll lose the grilled flavor.

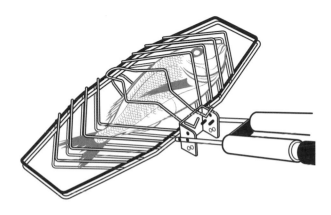

If you're feeling adventurous, you can wrap the fillet in something—a few pieces of bacon or prosciutto—and tie it up with raw twine, or bake it by placing it on a short plank of wood, setting it to one side, away from the hottest coals and covering the grill until the fish flakes to the touch. (Just make sure your wood is unvarnished and untreated, or you'll render your fish inedible.)

262 **What if I want to grill a bigger piece of meat?**

Slow cooking is the skill that separates the grilling gourmet from the weekend burger pusher. By turning your grill into an outdoor oven, you can cook up whole chickens, spareribs, or an entire pork shoulder.

Once you have a full chimney starter's coals burning steadily, separate the coals into two piles at the sides of the fire grate and fashion a drip pan from a piece of foil for the center of the grate. Put the lid on your grill with the lid's vents half closed, and leave the bottom vents open. This will give you about an hour's burn. On a gas grill, make sure the heat is kept low.

Natural lump charcoal, which is made from trees and only trees, is a good idea for any grilling you do, but especially for long-form grilling. The fume-free natural coals offer a distinct advantage, because after an hour, if your meat has not reached its desired temperature, you can replenish the heat by adding natural lump charcoal without the food tasting like the petroleum binders found in regular briquettes.

263 **How do I cook a perfect medium-rare steak?**

Take the steak out of the refrigerator half an hour before you want to serve it and sprinkle it liberally with salt and pepper on both sides. Preheat the oven to 450°F, and while it's warming, heat an oven-safe

cast-iron skillet over a medium-high flame. Wait a minute, then push a half-inch slice of butter around the pan until the butter is melted and bubbling. Sear the steak on one side for two minutes, then turn it over and sear the other side. Turn off the flame, put both the steak and

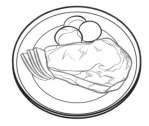

pan in the oven, and turn the oven off. Wait fifteen minutes.

Remove the steak from the pan and let it sit on a cutting board to rest and finish cooking. Wait about five to ten minutes to let the juices move back into the meat, then slice perpendicular to the grain of the steak and serve.

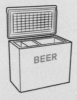

EXPERT WITNESS

264 HOW DO I BREW MY OWN BEER?

IAN McCONNELL
head brewer, Sixpoint Craft Ales, Brooklyn, New York

"The thought of making your own may sound intimidating, but trust me, it's completely possible and fairly cheap. For about a hundred dollars you can buy a home-brewing kit, which contains grain, malt extract, two buckets, and a hydrometer for measuring dissolved sugars. You'll also need a six-quart stockpot, and the tools you need for bottling, which usually come with the kit. The beer you make with the kit won't be the best you've ever tasted, but it won't bother you, because you're not a connoisseur yet. You'll just be thrilled that you've made your own beer.

"Once you've made one batch and like it, you can step up to glass fermenters instead of the plastic buckets that came with your kit. You'll also want to substitute liquid yeast if you've been using dry—liquid is more pure and kicks off the fermentation better. After a few more tries, you'll start to geek out about different malts and making your own yeast cultures—you have a lot of time while the beer is fermenting and conditioning to read up on your new hobby.

"While any home brewer can tell you stories about exploding bottles or beer that never fermented, the real danger is getting lazy and losing interest: though the actual brewing only takes three or four hours, it can be a lot of work tending to things and keeping track of the process. But the biggest obstacle is thinking you need a lot of skill or space. Brewing beer is really quite simple. I made my first batch in the kitchen of the apartment I shared with two other guys."

265 **How do I make a reduction sauce?**

Any guy can guess his way through cooking a steak; accompanying it with a delicious sauce sets you apart. While the steak is resting, chop up a big clove of garlic. Now go back to your still-messy pan and fire up the heat again, this time to medium. Pour in a cup or so of whatever deep, meaningful red wine you're serving with the steak. Using the front edge of a spatula, scrape the bottom of the pan, mixing the leftover crud and juices into the wine. Toss in the garlic and a tablespoon of thyme, add a half inch of a stick of butter. Let the liquid boil off, stirring occasionally, for three to four minutes. Done. Pour it over the whole steak after you place it on a platter, or pour the sauce into a small pitcher and let guests administer it themselves.

266 **What do I make with steak if I don't have an hour to bake a potato?**

With the oven already at 450°F but before you cook your steak, take two or three Yukon potatoes and slice them lengthwise into eighths. Toss them with some olive oil and salt—coarse sea salt or kosher salt is best—and arrange them in a single layer on a baking sheet. Bake them for fifteen minutes, turn them with a spatula, and put them back in for another ten or so before you pop the steak in and turn off the heat.

267 **How do I slice vegetables the way chefs do on TV?**

Practice. Position your fingers like you are holding a small ball, with your fingertips bent inward. Hold the item you're chopping between

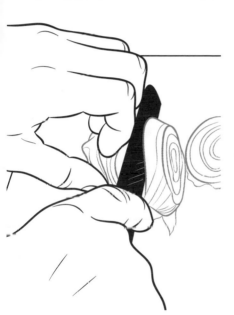

your thumb and forefinger and let the other fingers fall along the near face of the knife blade. As you lever the knife up and down, rocking it back and forth on an imag ined fulcrum about an inch back from the tip, push the item toward the blade. Use the fingers braced against the blade to guide the knife and protect your thumb and forefinger as you slice. Start slowly and build up speed as you gain confidence.

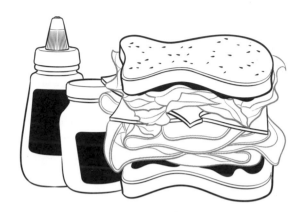

268 **What goes into making the perfect sandwich?**

The ingredients for the ultimate sandwich vary according to taste (and what happens to be in the refrigerator). Don't be afraid to experiment with flavors you've never combined before. But a few fundamentals need to be observed for the sandwich to come together.

▶ **THE BREAD** A chewy, crusty bread—a French baguette, hearty rye with or without caraway seeds, or a peasant loaf—is the proper platform on which to build your creation, to establish a formidable barrier against sogginess.

▶ **THE CONDIMENTS** When applying more than one, keep them segregated. In a traditional sammy put mustard on the bread surface closest to the meat, mayonnaise on the other slice. But don't stick to tradition: try salad dressing, olive oil, or horseradish.

Three classic grilled sandwiches

THE REUBEN Slather two slices of rye bread with Russian salad dressing, cover with corned beef, Swiss cheese, and sauerkraut. Grill for about three minutes a side in a lightly oiled or buttered pan, flipping once and pressing flat with the underside of a spatula.

THE ITALIAN Lightly brush peasant bread with olive oil, cover with sliced mozzarella and thinly sliced and seeded tomato. Add fresh basil, parsley, or pesto. Cook as above.

PEANUT BUTTER AND BACON Also known as the Elvis, this works best with whole wheat, slathered in peanut butter with two to four slices of bacon, grilled as above, minus the pressing. (The peanut butter will ooze out all over the pan.) For a more complex taste and a more filling meal, add sliced banana and drizzle with honey before topping with the bacon.

▶ **THE DRESSING** Lettuce lends the illusion of healthy greens, but its crispiness fades quickly as it absorbs oil. Spinach or sprouts fend off fats longer and seriously boost the nutritional value of the sandwich.

▶ **THE FILLING** Meat or cheese, sliced thin enough to see through, ideally brings its own flavor: be it cured, smoked, or peppered. Don't layer slices. Pick each one up by pinching it in the middle and place it gently onto the bread in a crumpled heap.

269 **How do I get the best meal from a vending machine?**

Think protein—those low-cal cookies are marketed as the healthy choice, but they won't stand up to your hunger. If there are bags of nuts, buy as many as you can eat. Peanut-brittle bars or those orange crackers with a thin line of peanut butter may be the next best thing. If nothing nutty is offered, make do with the least evil carbs: pretzels are fat-free and tasty, and baked chips, at least, skip much of the fat of the regular fried version.

270 **How do I carve a turkey?**

The honor of carving the bird at the holidays is usually reserved for the alpha male. When the knife falls to you, you want to have a plan. Here's a nontraditional but snazzy scheme you can execute with confidence and a surgeon's flair.

With the turkey's legs pointed away from you, take a sharp, medium-size knife and cut into the depression between one thigh and the body [a]. Gently pull on the leg as you slice [b], until the point of the knife finds the thighbone joint [c]. Cut through the joint to remove the leg, and divide the leg into the drumstick and thigh, again by cutting to one side of the joint [d].

Turn the thigh over, remove the bone running down its center [e]. Flip it back over and slice it in half widthwise [f]. Place these pieces on the serving platter.

Remove the wing in the same way, finding the joint as you pull back on the wing and cutting it away. Place the wing whole on the platter.

Repeat the entire process on the opposite side of the bird.

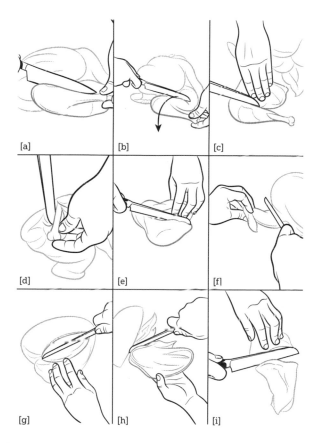

[a]

[b]

[c]

[d]

[e]

[f]

[g]

[h]

[i]

The breast is now fully exposed for carving. Find the shallow depression dividing the breast and slice the length of it [g] until the bird is in two large pieces [h]. Separate each breast from the breast-bone and slice it across its length in half-inch to one-inch chunks [i]. This makes for juicy, tender slices cut across the grain.

271 **How do I crack an egg?**

Give the side of the egg a sharp but gentle tap on the flat surface of the counter close to your pan or bowl [a]. (Using an edge will likely scatter bits of shell into your food.) Moving the egg over the bowl or pan, place the tips of your thumbs along each side of the crack you've made and gently pry the shell apart [b].

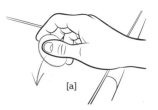
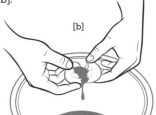

272 **How do I cook eggs?**

Even if you think you can't cook, you can certainly cook eggs. When your new squeeze asks, "How do you take your eggs?" be ready to offer any style she likes.

▶ **OMELET** Guys are prone to experimentation in the kitchen, which is why omelets are essential guy food. Dice, grate, or crumble Cheddar, Swiss, or goat cheese, sausage, bacon, or crabmeat, spinach, tomato, avocado, or scallions—anything you can imagine going into an omelet goes into one. (All raw meat should be cooked before you add it; you can also sauté your vegetables for just a minute before adding.) You can grate a little Swiss and leave it at that, as long as you have your fillings cut into small pieces and nearby.

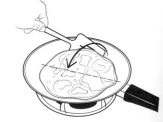

273 What are some classic cocktails I should know how to mix?

1 GIMLET If you're intimidated by the martini mixology, the gimlet is a pop fly: two parts gin to a half-part bottled lime juice. Serve as you would a martini: up and cold.

2 MANHATTAN Traditionally made as a bourbon martini; substitute blended whiskey or sweet red vermouth for dry white. Instead of olives, garnish with a maraschino cherry.

3 OLD-FASHIONED Put a teaspoon of sugar in the squat, heavy glass known as an old-fashioned and follow it with a dash of bitters. Fill the glass with ice cubes, then add an ounce of bourbon or blended whiskey. Top off with seltzer or sparkling water and garnish with a maraschino cherry, a wedge of orange, or both.

Heat a shallow pan over medium heat and coat the bottom with butter or olive oil. Prepare three large eggs as you would for scrambled eggs (see page 241), and pour them into the pan.

When the eggs are cooked on the bottom but are liquid on top, sprinkle your fillings in a line across the center of the eggs. Slip a spatula underneath the edge of the eggs and groove it around the perimeter to separate the cooking eggs from the pan. Now go back and flip one side then the other of the eggs over onto the center stripe of fillings. Place the omelet on a plate.

4

▶ **OVER EASY** Follow the
instructions for an egg sunny-side
up, but with a minute or so to go,
remove the pan from the heat,
tilting it away from you so that the
egg slides to the far side of the
pan. With a smooth upward flick of
your wrist, flip the egg backward
and over onto its opposite side.
(You can flip the egg with a spatula,
too, but where's the risk in that?)
After a minute, serve with salt and
pepper.

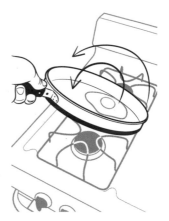

▶ **POACHED** Have a few eggs on hand, and more than your
usual measure of patience, since poaching eggs is a skill acquired
by practice. But once you have mastered this dying art, you'll be a
popular guest for breakfast.

Heat a pan of water slowly until bubbles begin to populate the
bottom and sides. Turn down the heat to keep the water just shy of
boiling. Break an egg into a small
teacup or a small heatproof bowl.
Place the lip of the teacup or
bowl against the side of the pan
just above the water. Quickly but
gently introduce the egg into the
water so that the egg doesn't
disperse and, most important, the
yolk doesn't break.

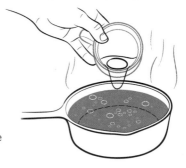

Wait three minutes or so, then tenderly raise the egg from the water using a slotted spoon or skimmer with a thin edge. The white of the egg should be opaque, and the yolk neither too runny nor too hard. Lay the egg gently on a slice of toast or English muffin, dab with butter and a few grains of pepper, and serve.

An inferior but serviceable poached egg can be made in the microwave. Break an egg into your teacup or bowl, add a couple of teaspoons of water, salt, and cover with a saucer. Microwave for three minutes.

▶ **SCRAMBLED** Scrambling eggs is one of those skills that's all in the wrist. In a small bowl, crack a couple of eggs, add a tablespoon of milk, a pinch of salt, and a half shake of pepper. Hold a fork firmly between your forefinger and thumb and, keeping your wrist loose, paddle the eggs with a motion that's half chop and half stir. Stop when the eggs are uniformly yellow and filled with air bubbles.

Heat your cast-iron pan or skillet over medium-low heat, adding a curl of butter or a dime-size spot of olive oil and swirling it around the pan.

Roll the eggs into the pan. Let the eggs set for nearly a minute before scraping the firm eggs gently while tilting the pan to allow the still-liquid eggs to spread evenly in the pan. Repeat until all the eggs are cooked. Remove from the pan while the eggs are still glossy, but not wet.

▶ **SUNNY-SIDE UP** Add a tablespoon of oil, butter, or bacon grease to a skillet set on medium heat. Let it warm and then crack an egg low over the pan and drop it in gently. Using a flexible spatula, separate any sticky spots from the pan. Let the egg bubble and pop from three minutes (loose yolk) to as long as five (solid yolk). Some cooks dip into the hot oil with a spoon and splash it onto the yolk for more flavor and a dash more heat. After transferring the egg to a plate, hit it with salt and pepper.

274 **What three easy meals can I learn to cook?**

No one expects you to be a master chef, so know that your first attempt to make a meal doesn't have to be perfect. You can also relieve the pressure by starting with one of these easy recipes.

▶ **PASTA ALFREDO** This meal requires you only to boil a box of pasta (fettuccine is traditional, but any form will do). Alfredo is quick and easy, as the other ingredients—grated Parmesan cheese, butter, milk or cream, and garlic—require no other cooking.

Heat plenty of water in a big pot until it's at a frenzied boil, and add a big pinch of salt and a pound of pasta. While it cooks, mince a garlic clove or two. When the pasta is soft all the way through but chewy, drain the water out of it in a colander. Put a half to a full stick of butter in the pot and dump the hot pasta on top and toss until every strand is coated. Add half a cup of milk or cream, the garlic, and half a cup of Parmesan. Crank as much pepper as you can stand, then toss everything together.

▶ **CHICKEN CURRY** This tomato-y Indian dish is passionately colorful and spicy. Serve it the first time you make dinner for someone you want to impress.

Five cool flicks from the sixties and seventies that every guy should know

1 | ***THE FRENCH CONNECTION*** Credited with the best car chase ever filmed, it stars Gene Hackman as Popeye Doyle, a cop sworn to putting an end to a heroin ring.

2 | ***THE CONVERSATION*** Hackman again, this time as a surveillance expert who gets burned by a client. It captures the post-Watergate era's paranoid mood.

3 | ***BONNIE AND CLYDE*** Warren Beatty as the 1930s bank robber and Faye Dunaway as his moll. In typical late-sixties fashion, the bad guys are the good guys, even if they're a little demented.

4 | ***CHINATOWN*** Jack Nicholson stars as a Los Angeles private eye who spends the entire movie figuring out he's been duped.

5 | ***THE GRADUATE*** Feeling lost after graduating from school? Meet Ben Braddock. The combination of Mike Nichols's witty direction and Dustin Hoffman's blank despair defined an era in the movies and young adulthood.

Buy two or three boneless chicken breasts, a twenty-eight-ounce can of whole tomatoes, a medium onion, a head of garlic, a piece of fresh ginger half the size of your thumb, a yellow onion, vegetable oil, a box of cloves and cinnamon sticks, curry powder, and rice. (If you can find basmati rice, use that.) Yogurt is optional.

Slice the chicken breasts into two-inch-wide chunks. Peel and slice the onion and then chop it, first in one direction, then turn your knife and chop again. Mince 3 or 4 cloves of garlic. Whittle the skin off the ginger with a grater, and grate the yellow flesh.

Make the rice by combining a cup of rice and one and a half cups of water in a small pot that has a lid. After bringing the contents to a vigorous boil, reduce the heat to a minimum and let the rice simmer with a lid on the pot for fifteen minutes.

Heat oil in a pot over medium heat. Toss in two cloves and a stick of cinnamon. When they begin to pop, add the onion and let the mixture sizzle about three minutes. Add the garlic, ginger, and two tablespoons of curry powder for another three minutes before throwing in the chicken.

While the chicken browns, chop the tomatoes roughly, then add them to the pot. Cover and turn down the heat until the liquid is just bubbling. Cook for five more minutes, or until the chicken is tender. Just before serving, add a dollop of yogurt and stir it in. Serve over rice.

▶ **SPINACH-AND-HAM QUICHE** Think of this as an omelet without the fancy flipping. Buy premade, uncooked pie shells, eggs, chunky ham slices, frozen spinach, a bag of grated Cheddar, a yellow onion, garlic, milk, and dried or fresh basil. You'll need an eight- or nine-inch pie pan if you're making your own crust (the foil one that comes with some premade pie shells will do, too).

Preheat the oven to 425°F. Unroll the pie shell and gently press it into the pan with the edges left up.

Microwave the frozen spinach in a bowl with a splash of water for four minutes while you chop the onion coarsely. Mince the garlic, and sauté with the onion for five minutes in a dab of oil. Add the microwaved spinach and a teaspoon of basil leaves, and sauté the whole thing until the liquid is gone.

Crack five eggs into a large bowl, add one cup of milk, and scramble.

Put half the spinach mixture in the pie shell. Sprinkle a cup of cheese on top, then sprinkle the rest of the spinach, and then the cheese again. Pour in the egg mixture.

Crimp the edges of the piecrust with your thumb and forefinger so it curls over the filling and put the whole deal into the oven. Immediately turn the oven down to 375°F and let the quiche cook for about thirty minutes. When the top is bubbling and getting brown, remove and let the quiche cool for five minutes before slicing like a pie and serving.

275 What's an easy recipe for an apple pie?

No one expects a guy to show up to a picnic or a dinner with a pie he made himself. Which is what makes the payoff so much greater than the effort involved.

Peel and quarter six Granny Smith apples, paring away the seeds and core and then halving the quarters and halving the eighths [a]. Put all the apples in a bowl along with a third of a stick of butter that you've diced up, two tablespoons each of lemon juice and flour, a teaspoon of cinnamon, and a half cup of honey [b]. Mix gently but thoroughly.

Unroll a premade piecrust and fit it into a pie pan, glass or metal. Pour the apple mixture on top and give a light shake to distribute the mixture evenly [c]. Unroll a second pie crust and lay it lightly over the top. (Bonus points: lay the second pie crust on a cutting board and slice it into long strips, then crisscross the strips in a loose lattice across the top of the pie.)

1
2
3
4
5
6

With a fork, gently crimp the two pie shells together around the edge to form a single ridge of crust around the pie's perimeter [d]. Use a fork to poke a few steam vents in the top piecrust.

Put the pie into an oven you've preheated to 425°F [e]. After about ten minutes, lower the temperature to 350°F and bake for another half hour. Serve warm and with a generous scoop of vanilla ice cream.

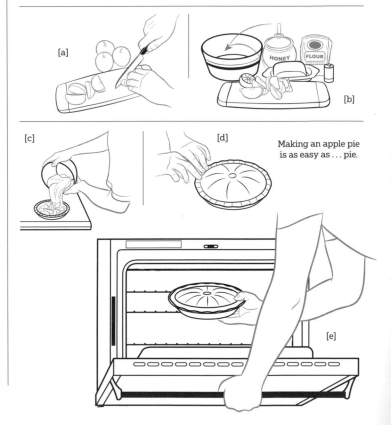

Making an apple pie is as easy as . . . pie.

THE HIGH LIFE

276 **How do I throw a cocktail party?**

The bare essentials of booze, something to eat, and a crowded room are a practically foolproof combination. What challenges every host is just how much of each to have.

Figure on two drinks per person for the first hour, then one for the rest of the party. The cheapest and simplest method is to nominate a theme cocktail—margaritas or, in sticky midsummer, gin and tonics. If you go with a full bar, count each bottle of hard stuff as fifteen drinks, and have two bottles of vodka and rum for every one of bourbon, Scotch, and gin, backed up with two liters of cola, seltzer, tonic, and orange juice. You'll also need a raft of beer and wine.

For hors d'oeuvres, you don't have to rush out for caviar. Buy frozen pigs-in-a-blanket from a bulk bargain store. Cook up a few frozen pizzas and slice them into finger-food-size squares, put out chips and store-bought dip, along with baby carrots. Note: If you have your party after dinner hours, the guests won't eat as much food.

As with your cocktails, you can also employ a theme for the party at-large. Hang strings of Chinese lanterns around your place and heat up frozen egg rolls and spring rolls as a nosh. If you have a yard, pitch a white canopy tent—inexpensive versions are available at the big-box hardware stores—and throw a Moroccan party, with candles in colored glasses, and hummus and pita for food.

277 **What does it take to be a good host?**

For the first half of the party, greet your guests and introduce them to one another. (Early arrivals are usually happy to be given an easy chore to finish while you man the floor.) Don't take coats, which bogs down the reception line. Instead, designate a place like a bed or a couple of large chairs for wraps and tell people to dump them there. Thank guests for any food or liquor they've brought and direct them to the bar, which has corkscrews in plain sight, or the kitchen, where you've left out extra serving bowls.

When the doorbell slows down, replenish your bar table and your hors d'oeuvres and other munchies, then circulate, keeping your eye out for isolated guests and introducing groups from work to your cousin or other personal acquaintances.

278 **How do I make punch for a party?**

An alcoholic punch that's strong enough for serious partiers and sweet enough for the occasional drinkers gives both groups a bonding experience. Here are two classic punches:

▶ **FRENCH 75** is the punch named for the World War I 75-mm howitzer used by the French army. Mix requires two bottles of champagne, a liter of cognac, and a liter of ginger ale.

▶ **FISHHOUSE PUNCH,** made by combining a bottle of dark rum, a liter each of brandy and club soda, and a cup each, or to taste, of peach brandy, lemon juice, and confectioners' sugar.

DIY

279 **How do I make the perfect dry martini?**

James Bond's habit of drinking very dry martinis ("shaken not stirred") established the cocktail as the suavely masculine choice. Bond, for the record, preferred vodka over gin in the Ian Fleming novels (and once asked for a gagging concoction of two parts gin, one part vodka, and a splash of a bitter wine flavored with quinine); a hipper model for the martini is this simple but effective recipe associated with Frank Sinatra.

Combine the gin and vermouth with several large ice cubes into a cocktail shaker (or any ample tumbler). Swirl them—neither shaking nor stirring—just until the shaker feels cold to the touch, but not long enough that ice melts into the spirits. Pour into a chilled glass whose inside you've smudged with a twist of lemon or an unpitted olive or two. Drink it before it gets warm.

The proportions of gin to white vermouth are a matter of historic debate, but as a baseline, start with two parts gin and one-half part dry vermouth. Less vermouth makes the martini drier: ratchet down the vermouth until you call it perfect.

GUYS' LIST ■

Meet the beer family

There are a million beers out there, but here's a list of the four main categories you need to know.

LAGER is a lighter, less alcoholic brew that hits the spot on a summer day or when you're thirsty. National brands like Bud or Miller are lagers, usually a very clean type of lager called pilsner, but in recent years a huge variety of local "craft" brewers have popped up to produce dense, flavorful beers all categorized as lagers. Lager is a versatile companion for food, whether you pair a pizza or chili with a dense "craft" brand or a lighter, mass-produced label with pasta alfredo.

ALES are more complex, more alcoholic, and in their most profound expression shade into the dark stouts. Their complexity isn't a function of their darker color, but of their heavy dose of hops, which lends a bitterness suitable to quiet conversation or silent contemplation. (Hops also extend the life of a beer, hence India pale ale, developed to withstand the voyage from Britain to India.)

STOUT is a barley-rich brew that runs from dry, extremely dark, and relatively low-alcohol brands to knock-your-socks-off Imperial stout to sweet cream stout and smooth oatmeal stout. Dry stout is perfect for fish, especially shellfish, and sweet dishes like chocolate cake at a birthday party. Cream stout goes with a hearty stew.

WHEAT Although this variety was almost unknown in the United States a few years ago, there is a growing competition between Belgian-style wheats—fruity and spicy—and clean German weizen, also known as "white" beer. Belgian wheats make for a nice sip before dinner, while the German variety is a good way to settle the tummy at the end of a night.

BEER

280 **How cold should I keep beer?**

You might have noticed mass-production beer commercials advertising the importance of drinking their product at frigid temperatures. But not all beer is meant to be drunk dead cold. A craft beer and any dark beer are made to be served in the low 40°F range, whereas a national brand pilsner with a lighter flavor and more carbonation is designed to be served in the mid-30s range. (For this reason, too, a more complex, darker beer is the one to buy if you're going mobile with no or little refrigeration.) You don't have to get two refrigerators to satisfy these requirements: store your light beers and other mass-production staples on the bottom shelf toward the back, and craft beers in the door, where the fridge is always a bit warmer.

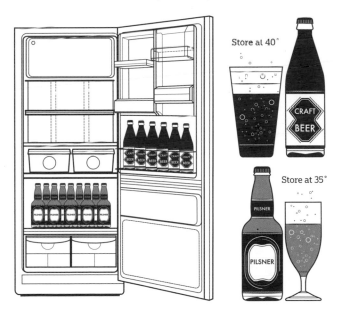

Store at 40°

Store at 35°

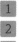

281 Should I always drink beer out of a glass?

Not necessarily. Craft brews should be poured into a glass to release the flavor and allow you to sniff the beer's aroma. Mass domestics aimed at pure refreshment and formulated with a high level of carbonation may be sipped directly from a can or bottle, which keeps the beer cooler and fizzier.

282 How do I serve the hard stuff?

Hard liquor's popularity is rising again, especially among young people. If you are buying only one bottle of hard liquor to have on hand, it should be a quality vodka, which for some time has been the most popular spirit, and which mixes with almost anything you have in the fridge to make a cocktail, including Red Bull and heavy cream.

But a guy should know his booze and keep on hand a few poisons to pick from.

▶ **BOURBON** Known these days mostly as the stuff of mint juleps, America's only 100 percent homegrown whiskey used to be ubiquitous. Sweeter than Scotch and in many minds less sophisticated, bourbon has undergone rebranding of late as a highly aged sipping whiskey. Bourbon's close relative, Tennessee whiskey, also made from a corn sour mash, is double-filtered through charcoal before barrel aging.

HOW DO I DRINK IT? Look for "center-cut" bottlings or anything aged over a decade to drink neat. But old-schoolers see nothing

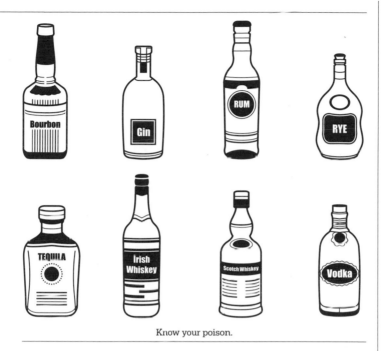

Know your poison.

wrong mixing a bar brand in Manhattans, whiskey sours, or simply with the barest drop or two of water, over ice.

▶ **GIN** Addictively fresh and summery light, the national spirit of Great Britain is a grain alcohol flavored with the aromatic juniper berry. Once nearly buried in its fusty Brit tradition, gin is now back on the map thanks to the resurgence in martini consumption over the past decade.

HOW DO I DRINK IT? When it comes to martinis—gin slightly sweetened with vermouth—the answer is very carefully. This is all the more true when the delivery system is candied up as an "appletini" or "crantini." Simpler measures are the gimlet, or, on a summer evening, a gin and tonic, which does a better job of diluting the gin.

▶ **RUM** Its Caribbean origin and connections to British privateers has unfortunately caused rum to be marketed with Jolly Rogers and strange flavorings. It's a shame, since white rum can be quite refreshing and dark rum is subtle and contemplative. Like gin, rum rewards an extra few bucks to get the good stuff.

HOW DO I DRINK IT? Anything vodka can do rum can do better: mix with orange juice, mush up with mint and sugar to make a mojito, or with soda or tonic water.

▶ **TEQUILA** Famed for its near-druglike effects, this Mexican spirit distilled from the agave cactus has made its own bid recently for connoisseur treatment, with first white, unaged tequilas being replaced by barrel-aged gold versions, then gold replaced by añejo at the top of the tequila fashion chain.

HOW DO I DRINK IT? Margaritas, almost the sole tequila drink for years, are giving way slowly to direct consumption of the aged, premium brands on the rocks. A tequila sunrise is so old-school many bartenders don't know how to make it (with grenadine), but it's sweetly delicious.

▶ **VODKA** The most popular hard liquor is extremely versatile, lending a refreshing bite to juices from cranberry to orange, and mixing companionably with tonic water. Once favored by drunks because it leaves little alcohol trace on the breath, vodka retains a reputation for stealth consumption in the belief that it won't give you a hangover. It will.

HOW DO I DRINK IT? In a martini, screwdriver, Bloody Mary, cosmopolitan, and countless other drinks.

Whiskies

▶ **BLENDED WHISKEY** Batches of whiskies made from a variety of grains are mixed to produce the smoothest, most drinkable brew. If not specified, "whiskey" refers to blended, and most to one of the better blendeds that hail from Canada.
HOW DO I DRINK IT? As a lighter alternative to bourbon in whiskey sours or old-fashioneds.

▶ **IRISH WHISKEY** The original whiskey, it's a blend of distillates of corn and malted and unmalted barley, and distinguished from its Scottish younger cousin by keeping the malt away from smoke, preserving the grain's sweeter toasted flavor.
HOW DO I DRINK IT? On the rocks, neat.

▶ **RYE** Made almost identically to bourbon, American rye is distilled from the same grain that goes into rye bread, and has the same spicy, dry twist.
HOW DO I DRINK IT? Substituted for bourbon in cocktails like a Manhattan, it renders the drink less sweet.

▶ **SCOTCH** For sheer variety, history of serious connoisseurship, and pure mystique, malt whiskey made in Scotland rules all other whiskeys. It's worth developing a taste for bar Scotch simply to be able to appreciate the single malts—whiskeys made from a single batch of fermented barley each with their own controlled, peculiar character—that are treasured and traded like fine wine among enthusiasts.

HOW DO I DRINK IT? While there's no crime in splashing soda water and ice into a bar Scotch, a single malt should be sipped straight, no ice, with a nibble of smoked salmon on crackers or even a few squares of chocolate.

283 **How do I order liquor at a bar?**

The bartender will be more likely to return to you promptly if you order efficiently. Don't start ordering until you know what everyone in your group wants and order according to type of beverage if you can manage it, for example, "Two Miller Lites, a white wine, and a Fuzzy Navel." It also pays to know the bartender's lingo for how you want your drink served.

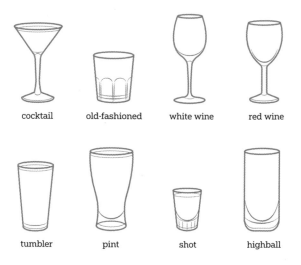

cocktail   old-fashioned   white wine   red wine

tumbler   pint   shot   highball

▶ **NEAT** The drink will be served in an old-fashioned or whiskey glass at room temperature. Whiskies are the most common liquors drunk neat.

▶ **ROCKS, OR ON THE ROCKS** The drink will come over ice in an old-fashioned glass or a tall glass called a highball.

▶ **SHOT** An ounce or ounce and a half of straight liquor or a fruity blend, served in a shot glass.

▶ **UP, OR STRAIGHT UP** The drink will be chilled by being shaken or stirred in a cocktail shaker and strained into a glass with no ice. Martinis, cosmopolitans, and sometimes margaritas are served up.

284 **How do I tip a bartender?**

If you've run a tab on a credit card, simply add a tip of 15 to 20 percent when you close your tab, as you would do for a waiter or waitress. If you are paying cash as you go—or if you want to ensure prompt service on a busy night—leave a dollar on the bar (two if you're in a big group) every time you get served. Don't be shy about pushing your tip toward the inside edge of the bar so the bartender has no doubt whose money it is. True, by the end of the night the bartender will have collected the price of an entire drink from you, but he or she knows this as well as you, and may well kick it back to you with a free round.

1
2
3
4
5
6

285 **How do I drink a flaming shot?**

Blow on the flame or cover it briefly with a small plate to extinguish it before knocking your shot back. Any attempt to get the shot into your mouth while it's ignited will almost certainly result in pouring flaming liquid onto your clothes or hair.

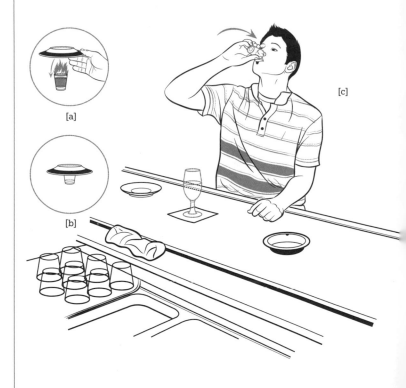

[a]

[b]

[c]

286 **How do I drink and not get drunk?**

Your liver can handle one drink an hour—one wine, one beer, or one standard cocktail—without backing up and making you tipsy. But since nursing a drink for that long can make you look like a stick-in-the-mud, diplomats and others who attend receptions as a profession 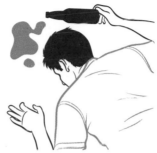 have developed strategies to look like they are drinking more than they are. Alternate your cocktails with something that looks like one—for instance, club soda with a twist can pass for a gin and tonic.

Another strategy is to order something intense, like a single-malt Scotch or the densest beer on tap, which forces you (and satisfies you) to sip it while everyone else chugs.

287 **How do I manage a hangover?**

You went out and had a crazy time and now the next day you're paying for it. Try to use as many of the following seven tips as you can the next time you're nursing a hangover and you'll be as good as new in no time.

▶ **THE BEST OFFENSE AGAINST A HANGOVER IS A GOOD DEFENSE.** Before heading out to the bar or party, down two aspirin or Advil to prevent the blood coagulation that causes headache. As you drink, and before going to bed, drink generous amounts of water to counteract the dehydrating effects of alcohol.

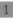

Sports drinks with no caffeine are good for replacing electrolytes you've flushed away.

▶ **SLEEP AS LONG AS YOU CAN.** The only tried-and-true antidote to overindulgence is time. You might as well be asleep while your body metabolizes the alcohol and rebalances.

▶ **RESTORE YOUR NUTRIENTS.** You may not feel hungry, but nibbling a banana, apple, or taking a vitamin pill will bring your potassium and magnesium back up to par.

▶ **CAFFEINATE.** Coffee, dark soda, or tea will help constrict the capillaries in your head to reduce the headache and "big head" feeling.

▶ **COOL YOUR EYES.** Wrap ice cubes or slightly wet tea bags in a cloth and apply them to your eyes for ten to fifteen minutes to reduce telltale puffiness.

▶ **GET A LITTLE EXERCISE.** Help your body pump out the poisons by getting in a workout or taking a little walk.

▶ **MAKE AMENDS.** Call someone you think you might have kissed, told off, or thrown up on and apologize. It won't make you feel better physically, but you'll stop feeling like an ass and maybe get to have a laugh about your behavior.

288 **How do I navigate a formal place setting?**

The dazzling array of silverware at a formal meal can look confusing when you first sit down, but the formula is easy: as each course arrives, simply use the outermost utensil and work to the middle. You can also generally identify your utensils by size and placement: The largest fork and knife are for the main course [a]. The slightly smaller fork [b] is the salad fork, and the smallest, often placed above your plate, is for dessert [c]. The soup spoon is identifiable by its large, round bowl [d]. Smaller and smallest spoons will be for dessert and coffee, respectively [e]. A butter knife will be small, blunt, and often will appear on your bread plate [f].

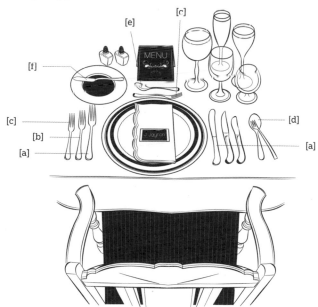

289 **How do I signal to the waiter that I'm finished eating?**

When you've finished a course, place your used fork turned down slightly to the right of the top rim of your plate, at an angle, along with any other utensils you're ready to have taken away [a]. (Never lay any utensil on the tablecloth once you've picked it up.)

Your napkin also operates as a signal. Put it on your lap when you sit down and unfold it. (No flapping it like a checkered flag to the side or tucking it under your chin—you won't be slurping in a class joint. In a casual restaurant, tossing your tie over your shoulder is acceptable.) When you leave the table and intend to return, place the napkin on your chair back [b]. (The waiter in a fancy joint may replace it before you get back.) A napkin on the table, like a white flag, says you are quitting the field and not coming back.

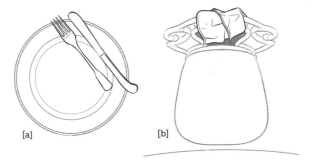

[a]   [b]

5

Birds and Bees

Romance for guys is a conundrum. She wants you to observe the rules, say the right things, make the right moves—only to tell you that you had her at hello. Why not just cut to the chase?

FOREPLAY

290 **What's the best pickup line?**

Studies show—and here's a field of inquiry worth its grant money—
that the most effective way to make initial contact with someone
you're attracted to is to give your name and ask hers, as in: "Hi, my

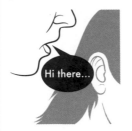

name is __, what's yours?" Not only won't it
creep her out the way a rehearsed come-on
will, she'll also be impressed with your confidence. Have another comment in reserve
for the next step, optimally having to do
with the event or the surroundings, not how
bodacious her snoobs are.

Hi there...

291 **How do I start a conversation?**

Context is everything. Involve an attractive stranger in your immediate situation in a way that exhibits your best features: at a store
counter, ask for help picking out a gift (which signals your generos-
ity and thoughtfulness), question the sanity of the artist at a gallery
(independence of mind, humor), etc. The approach allows her to give
her opinion as well.

292 **How do I flirt?**

Charm isn't something everyone has. Maybe you get tongue-tied, or
you can't think of what to talk about. Never mind. Flirting is more
about listening than it is about talking. Stop trying to be interesting

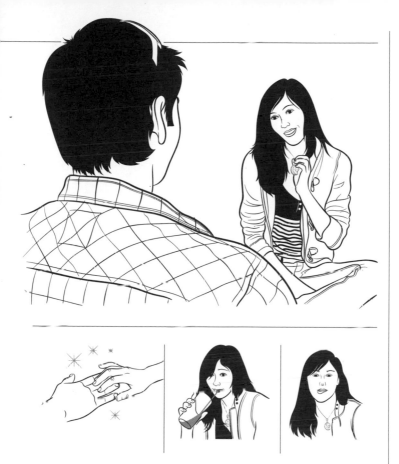

and be interested. Ask the other person to tell you more. You'll likely be asked to talk about yourself in return—a topic you can handle. Be self-deprecating without resorting to sarcasm.

Second, because flirting is all about subtext, it doesn't much matter what you talk about. It's in the way you smile, lean in to hear her over the music, or simply keep her gaze even when the conversation has stopped. Be alert for her subtext, too: playing with jewelry, friendly touches, mysterious looks, or unconscious hair twirling could be signs of interest.

Nine ideas for great first dates

ART MUSEUM The quiet surroundings and focus on what's on the walls allows you to spend time getting used to how your date moves and looks (and vice versa). Remember to develop an opinion about the art, too. Pick a specific exhibit (to keep the visit short), and go for coffee to talk about it.

TAKE A HIKE A date who likes the outdoors will be put at ease at a local nature preserve or nearby upland trail—don't stray too far from civilization. The exertion of a hill or two will excuse any awkward gaps in conversation, and a little hard breathing is also pleasantly suggestive.

TOURIST ATTRACTION Visit the local restored farm or the Native American burial ground or whatever site the two of you haven't seen since the school field trip. Bring your sense of humor.

GO BOWLING The goofiness of this classic pastime allows you to subtly show off your strength, and to drink beer, and gives her the chance to claim a place in your heart when she beats you.

293 **How do I make my move?**

The longer you wait, the more dramatic the move, and the more nervous you'll get. Start small, touching her on the arm or shoulder during a laugh. Tap her leg briefly while making a point. In the split second you touch, you can sense how she reacts. If she pulls away, you're not invited to go further, at least that evening. If your new friend is fine with that and continues the flirting behavior, pull back, but look forward to a more intimate touch when you're alone. On the walk home, you can try an arm around the shoulders or tangling your fingers.

CHILD'S BIRTHDAY PARTY
The innocence of your niece or nephew's games-and-cake get-together can be the perfect tone for the right girl, and the presence of a mix of other adults will keep the burden of conversation light. Contrast with a few stiff drinks afterward.

ROAD TRIP Time in the car means some heavy talking time, so keep any trek to a nearby city or activity under an hour. But getting out of your habitual environs will make even an ordinary movie or meal a little special.

MINIATURE GOLF You won't get points for originality, but the light competition, amusement-park atmosphere, and the chance to observe each other is what makes this a first-date tradition.

GO TO CHURCH Not a service, necessarily, but an organ or choral concert in an ornate house of worship, complete with candlelight and shadows, has an unmistakably sexy vibe.

SPORTS EVENT Nab two tickets to a high-level game, especially one that offers plenty else to do—a great food court or halftime show. Be relaxed about walking around the premises or leaving early. And if she wants to stay to see who wins, you'll know she's a winner.

The next area you want to make contact with is the lips, but if you're still unsure where the evening's headed, place your hip bone gently against the other party's. If the contact is welcomed, you have a green light to go further.

294 **What do I write in my profile on an Internet dating service?**

Read over a few profiles, noting the phrases and thoughts that recur with scandalous frequency, then avoid them. Don't announce your

1
2
3
4
5
6

search for "a woman who looks as good in jeans as she does in a black dress." Don't say you "love the city and all it has to offer," or that you like "walks on the beach." You want to stand out.

OLD SCHOOL

295 How do I ask someone for a date?

These days a guy has so many convenient technologies to work with—e-mail, IM, texting, social networking sites—that a face-to-face request to go out with someone seems as formal as a marriage proposal. The virtual ask, it's true, has a suitable neutrality; you don't want the moment to feel overwrought or climactic. But that same neutrality makes it easier for your prospective date to take a pass. Sometimes the best argument for a guy is that he had the balls to ask in person.

In that spirit, you don't want to be too gimmicky or indirect. Introduce the idea and quickly state your purpose, along the lines of "Hi, I really enjoyed meeting you the other day, and I'm wondering

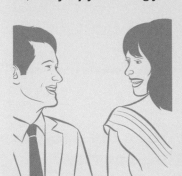

if you'd like to have dinner this weekend." Don't be afraid to show a little nervousness; the object of your attentions will be unsettled as well, and why not? What better way to begin a romance than with two thumping hearts?

If you're not likely to bump into each other, much the same note may be struck on a phone call. Don't start an e-mail chain or a text exchange and get distracted. Give your full attention, and be prepared to be witty and charming.

The best way to do that is to talk sincerely about yourself. You won't impress anyone by being cocky or boastful. Talk about your family; let the world know you like to hang with your kid sister. Be specific about the books you read, the movies you like, and music you listen to. Balance your list of requirements and the amount of information you provide. This gives the impression that you're as concerned with being a decent date as you are with finding one.

Be subtle about sexual expectations. There are code words that indicate your willingness without being demanding. The word "sensual" implies that your happiness includes sex but is not the whole reason for getting connected. Your agenda is clear without being graphic if you say, "I'm not in a hurry to find The One, but I'm not opposed to it."

Lastly, be truthful, especially about your looks. Pick a recent and representative photograph of yourself. If you misrepresent yourself online, your dates will never trust you about anything.

296 Where should I arrange a meeting with someone I met online?

This is what the modern rash of coffee shops are made for. Once you've made contact through the dating site, a couple of e-mails or phone calls to arrange a meeting are enough—don't talk the romance to death before it's started. Find a coffee shop in your contact's zip code and suggest you meet there. Or you can grab dinner or a drink. Be flexible and feel each other out. Don't take it personally if your match is nervous about meeting or actually says the words "ax murderer": the prospect of meeting a stranger with sex on his mind goes against what many of us were taught from an early age. Protracted stalling, however, should set off alarms; there's more going on than you want to know about, and you'll likely end up wasting your time.

If you haven't seen each other's picture (and really if someone doesn't have a picture these days that should also set off alarms), make sure you're in contact that day to find out how to recognize each other, and to exchange cell-phone numbers in case someone has to cancel at the last minute. (It's not fun being stood up, especially on the first-meeting date.)

297 **How do I play the virtual field?**

As in any other form of dating, honesty is required. Inform the person that you're not locking yourself in—"I'm new at this and I'm not dating anyone exclusively yet"—does the trick. Keep your signals clear by contacting your matches only when you invite them out. A rush of texts and phone calls gives the impression you're investing in the relationship, and when the wires go silent again, it will feel like a betrayal even if you've stated your agenda at the outset.

298 **How do I handle a date?**

The first date is the hardest, requiring both parties to dedicate an entire evening to a proposition that may end in (a) boredom, (b) rejection, or (c) life-altering change. Here are some steps that will reduce the stress:

Five great starter jazz albums

▶ *BLUE TRAIN* (1960) John Coltrane's 1957 debut as a bandleader after his long tutelage under Thelonious Monk and Miles Davis is relatively quiet, but promises his next steps.

▶ *COUNT BASIE AT NEWPORT* (1957) Ripping blues with an introduction to Lester Young on sax and Joe Williams's vocals amid the stylings of the Basie band.

▶ *ELLA IN BERLIN* (1960) Cosmopolitan, funny, visceral, ineluctable: the girl can flat-out sing.

▶ *KIND OF BLUE* (1959) Miles Davis leads a smoky, thoughtful, wide-open improvisation dreamed up by legendary pianist Bill Evans, who plays on most of the tracks.

▶ *THE SHAPE OF JAZZ TO COME* (1959) Ornette Coleman's warbling sax neatly presages the deep end of jazz in the 1960s, when genius tips into structured chaos.

▶ **HAVE AN ITINERARY IN MIND** Keep the date casual, but not so casual that you have to improvise. Take charge and explain what you have in mind before you get together or as you meet. It's also good to have a backup plan: if she's a vegetarian and you bet everything on eating at a steak house, the relationship may stall right there.

▶ **GIVE BOTH PARTIES AN OUT** Meet for drinks or coffee near a restaurant you're familiar with. If things go well, suggest that you keep the conversation going over dinner. If the conversation is like pulling teeth, you can pay the tab and say good night.

▶ **CREATE A BUFFER** If you're nervous about what you'll talk about, hit a movie so you can get comfortable together without having to talk. If you'd like to lower the stakes more, invite your love interest to go on a group date.

▶ **PASS THE MIKE** Talking too much, especially about yourself, is the death knell for a date. Pick a common occurrence—your date taking a sip of her drink or the jukebox striking up a new tune—and change the subject by asking a question every time it happens. Keep sarcasm, complaints, and foul language to a minimum.

299 **How do I pick up someone in a bar?**

When it comes to seduction, alcohol is a guy's best friend. Therefore a bar is the time-honored starting point for a one-night stand. But a bar isn't the only place: your odds go up in a place where women outnumber men—bookstores, museums, art galleries, and retail outlets, and there are even substitutes for booze. One of these is confidence. Instill some in yourself before you go on the prowl by treating yourself to an expensive haircut, buy a new piece of clothing, and wear an outfit you know you look good in. Pamper yourself.

She will likely spot your intentions a mile off. If you're rebuffed, move on but don't give up. A woman who is dismissive or unsettled by your attention at first may find that your pursuit was the most entertaining thing about the evening, or may get jealous to see you flirt with another.

Lastly, don't forget to equip yourself with a condom. Lack of protection can be a last-minute deal breaker. When you're ready to go, decide on a location (your place? her place? the bathroom stall at the back of the bar?) and get to it.

300 **What do I do when a one-night stand is over?**

The sex was great. Is breakfast really going to be better? If your partner invites you to stay, but you'd rather not, state that you're flattered—you should be, after all—and promise to call. A cheesy line about having a meeting in the morning or your mother coming over

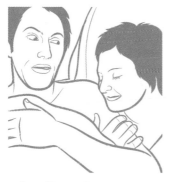

early to measure for curtains is just going to deepen the impression that you're a heel.

If you brought her to your digs, allow her to leave with her dignity intact. Offer her something to wear—an old shirt, say—and a cup of coffee. Disguise impatience with a show of concern—"You okay to drive?" or "Let me call you a cab"—

and you'll start the conversation with the appropriate touch of grace.

Before you rush to clear out or show her the door, take a moment to consider whether you want to see her go. You've already gotten over the toughest hurdle; a friendship, at least, may be on the other side.

301 **How do I have a fun buddy?**

A friend with benefits trusts you enough to be a casual lover. You share interests and go places together. Having sex is an extension of

1
2
3
4
5
6

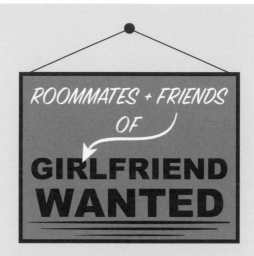

EXPERT WITNESS

302 CAN I DO THE ROOMMATE SWITCH?

LYNN HARRIS
cocreator of Break Up Girl blog

"Pencil the roommate in for never. Or at least not as long as they're still roommates. If you're interested in the non-roommate friend of someone you've dated heavily for six months—and we're talking really interested, as in 'Could Be the One' interested, not 'Could Be Cute, I Guess' interested—you have to wait at least twice that long before making your move. And that move is: mentioning your interest first to your ex. 'I know this is incredibly awkward,' you might say, 'but I wanted to let you know that I was planning on asking out so-and-so.' Alternative: if things are already kind of moving and shaking with the friend, agree not to tell the ex until you know for sure it's a thing. This way, if it fizzles, you won't (potentially) have to hurt the ex's feelings—or friendship—for nothing."

your other recreational activities. If you want to recruit an existing friend for this kind of arrangement, the sex will happen naturally, but talk about it afterward. "You know me," you might say, "I'm not ready to have a full-time relationship, but I sure enjoyed what happened. Let's just play it by ear."

All benefits have a cost. Check in with yourself often about your feelings. Realize that you may not be the only buddy on the other person's list. And be prepared to step aside if your buddy meets someone else and you don't have a better offer. If you feel your heart getting engaged, you need to rewrite the contract or get out of the deal.

303 How do I talk about my sexually transmitted disease with a potential partner?

If you're a healthy guy who happens to be living with an STD, you unfortunately have to have the talk with everyone you want to take to bed. Here are a few pointers to make it a little easier.

▶ **WHEN** The earlier you talk about what you've got, the more time the other person has to adjust. After all, she was thinking about sex, too, and needs not only to digest new information but to reimagine what that sex will be like. The closer you are to taking off your clothes, the less likely your relationship will recover.

▶ **HOW** Don't present yourself as a statistic. Frame the facts as a narrative: a very G-rated but truthful version of how you contracted the disease (without betraying anyone's privacy or causing more hurt: if you got the disease while cheating, deal with it as a separate

5
6

issue), how long you've had it, what the symptoms are. Once you talk about yourself, tell the facts about risks of transmission and treatments. Be prepared to answer a lot of questions.

▶ **WHERE** In person, when nobody else is around. Take a long walk in a solitary place or somewhere your partner has the freedom to leave if she needs space.

304 **When should I send flowers?**

There are not a lot of rules about giving flowers, since they are appreciated almost any way they are offered. Showing up with flowers when you pick her up for a date indicates your excitement in a manfully tacit fashion. Sending flowers to a young lady's office creates a satisfying stir, and provokes questions about who sent them—thereby signaling that you're glad to acknowledge your new relationship.

Flowers are not a substitute for saying you're sorry. Apologies should be delivered in words, preferably in person or in a handwritten note. Hiding behind a bouquet is neither straightforward nor particularly manly. Once you've denounced your behavior properly, it's fine to send a bouquet to show your sincerity.

305 **What kind of flowers should I send?**

You can't go wrong with roses, but don't hesitate to send other blooms, each of which has its own meaning. Here's a quick phrase book for the sentiment you're feeling and the flowers that match it:

- ▶ **Praising beauty** Oleander, orchids, magnolia, white camellias
- ▶ **New love** Pink roses
- ▶ **Desire** Orange roses
- ▶ **Passion** Red camellias, red roses
- ▶ **Unrequited love** Daffodils, red carnations
- ▶ **Remember me** Forget-me-nots, pink carnations, yellow roses
- ▶ **Secret love** Gardenias, white roses
- ▶ **Friendship** Mixed chrysanthemums, iris
- ▶ **Believe me** Red tulips, gladiolas

GETTING SERIOUS

306 **How do I tell if a relationship has legs?**

When you've met someone exciting and are spending enough time in close contact to be drinking in her pheromones, you tend to overlook things that spell trouble for a relationship. Enjoy getting to know a new person, but once you've come down to earth a little, it's a good idea to take a look at how much potential there is. Consider general compatibility and how you match up on such important topics as these:

▶ **FAMILY** Is she unable to make a move without asking her mother? Or is her independence from her parents closer to estrangement? Either way, you need to be able to live in her family system.

▶ **LEISURE TIME** Is she a homebody? A social butterfly? There's nothing wrong with either personality type, but if the two of you have different images of the perfect evening, you may see less of each other than the affair can handle.

▶ **MONEY** You want to own a house before you marry; she lets tomorrow take care of itself. Or you shower people with gifts, while she can't bring herself to spring for a bag of groceries for the weekend share. If you don't trust each other with your wallets, your mistrust will bleed into other parts of your romance.

▶ **POLITICS** Do you agree on major issues? Or if you don't, are you able to have constructive discourse? Are your worldviews compatible?

307 **How do we stop arguing?**

Every relationship entails a little controversy, and nobody's perfect. Arguments that arise from idiotic behavior on one party's part or the other can usually be resolved with apologies, a period of quiet, and a dinner out. A wise man explained how he'd remained married for seventy-five years: "When she was angry, I kept my mouth shut."

Other arguments mystify us: we find ourselves repeatedly grumbling about the same stuff every few months, and we're disgruntled for days afterward. Relationship experts say that romantic attraction is partly based on family dynamics: when we blow up repeatedly over the same perceived slight, we may be acting out the dramas of our childhood. At that moment you're yelling at someone not in the room. There's no sure way to tell which kind of argument you're having—if one party blurts out, "You always treat me like this!" or flies into a rage while the other looks on confused but calm, experts say, you've hit one of these tender spots. The best insurance is to stay alert to the baggage you bring to the relationship, and keep it separate from day-to-day disagreements.

308 What if my girlfriend doesn't want me to be friends with my exes?

First, make sure this ex is a friend worth fighting for: if you don't have a good reason, your principled stand may start to sound as if you have unfinished business. But if your friendship is all that's at stake, protest, in as casual and light a tone as possible, that you had every chance to make things work out with your ex. Remind your girlfriend that you are no longer going out with that other girl for a reason—that it was never going to work out. Also be prepared with every good reason why you need your ex as a friend. She's been there for you through hard times. She's a friend of the family—whatever truthful reasons you have.

309 How do I break up with someone?

It's going to hurt no matter what, but you have a responsibility to limit the sting. Do the deed at the other person's place if possible, where they are comfortable and you won't have to fidget through dessert, or offer her the ride home from hell.

Be honest, or as close to honest as you can get. Say you have had a great few months but just aren't in it for the longer haul. Make sure you are heard—your reasons are important—and return the favor by listening to her response, but don't argue or open a new can of worms. Nod, sigh with regret, and leave.

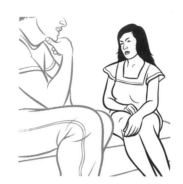

Finally, be careful what you wish for: the "cooler" she is about it, the more you'll wonder if she liked you at all.

310 **What do I do about my friend's obnoxious girlfriend?**

Let her be his problem, at least at first. At the beginning of a relationship, a couple spends the bulk of its time on planet Them, and you likely won't see much of the guy for a while anyway. The more intense the dose he gets of her, the sooner he'll see what you do. Or she may cool out as she gets more comfortable with you and the idea that she can share him with friends without losing him. (Consider, too, whether what you really object to is not her personality but her claim on his time.)

Love is mysterious, however; you may never understand his attraction and she may never change. Resist any temptation to cause strife between them. Your evil plot is prone to backfire and result in a serious break in your friendship. Instead, ask him to come out for guys' nights or to sporting events. Listen closely when he talks about her to gain some insight into what he likes about her: what you see as obnoxious he might view as spunk. Perhaps you'll come to see her as good for him. Regardless, keep in mind that despite your distaste for her, what's good for your pal should be your chief concern.

311 **How do I ask a woman to marry me?**

Pick a spot where you'll know you won't be interrupted, but don't worry too much about the perfect locale: the proposal itself will make that place special.

Similarly, let the gravity of the moment itself provide the drama; you need not contrive a special effect, like burying the ring in the oysters Rockefeller or arranging for a band to strike up the moment she says yes. These are memorable, but it's quite enough to tell her honestly and plainly why it's time she and you tied the knot—your love for her should play largely in your rationale—and pop the question in so many words: Will you please marry me?

Some women will want an engagement ring of a particular size and cut, others consider one an antifeminist declaration that you are her property. But consider your own feelings about laying down two months' salary (the ring budget recommended by wedding mavens)

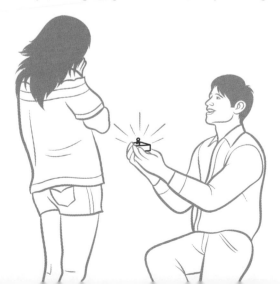

1
2
3
4
5
6

and then come up with a plan that will please both of you. Or, instead of a ring, hand over tickets to a destination she's always wanted to go to (especially if the wedding date is not set or is two years off).

If you're the romantic type who needs to surprise her with a diamond, by all means do so. Just be certain that the ring can be exchanged and assure her that the two of you can return it for her dream stone. These days, the odds are you will probably discuss the ring with her before you shop for it, so you'll have an idea of what she wants. However you play it, every experience is an opportunity to understand your bride-to-be better.

TECHNIQUE

312 **What should the first kiss be like?**

The first kiss should be a thumbnail sketch of your lovemaking skills, not a survey of your arsenal. Gently and briefly kiss her with lips slightly parted at first, offering no tongue—you need not even make first contact on her mouth; a few pecks scattered around her cheek, neck, and forehead are a nice warm-up to intimate kisses on her lips. If you have the patience, let her be the one to extend one of your kisses into a more passionate smooch.

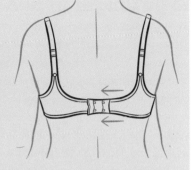

313 How do I undo a bra?

It's always best to let bras come off by mutual agreement. But if she clearly wants you to do the deed, you don't want to fumble it. First, determine where the clip is. In midhug, feel the back of her bra for a bumpy strip. If there's none, it's either around front or she's wearing a sports bra that comes off over her head.

Next determine whether the clasp is a classic hook and eye (you'll feel two or three small bumps under fabric) or a plastic S-clip (you'll feel a smooth plastic tab). If the clasp is in front, it is almost certainly a plastic S.

The basic action for the hook and eye is a gentle, sustained squeeze with your thumb and forefinger. Begin your squeeze with your fingers about an inch or more apart: the clasp will buckle up as you squeeze; as it does, rub the thumb and forefinger together like you are snapping. (Hint: the hooks are on the left, so put more pressure on that side.) The bra should pop open.

Plastic clasps, front or back, require a diagonal motion as you squeeze. Hook your forefinger underneath the clasp to guard against digging the clasp into her skin as you squeeze and release. All these techniques improve with practice. If you get it on the first try, don't let her see how surprised you are.

314 **What tricks can I use to go longer in bed?**

Every guy has his tricks to delay the onrushing inevitable, be it a meditative mantra or summoning a mental image of his high school gym teacher, but like many another problem, the best solution is exercise. Your only physical hope of controlling your ejaculation is to exercise the muscles behind your scrotum with a technique called the Kegel.

Here's how: alternately tense and relax the muscles behind your scrotum and forward of your butt. Do kegel reps as you lie in bed or while riding in the car. See how long you can hold the tension. Guys find that the more they can control those muscles, the longer they can hold off.

315 **Should I use erectile dysfunction drugs?**

Despite the white-haired gents dancing with their wives in the commercials, it's not unknown for younger guys to experience erectile dysfunction. More commonly, dudes take boner pills to see what spawned a billion pieces of junk mail. Different brands have different effects: some work as they enter the bloodstream; others only show their mettle when you are engaged in lovemaking activity. All of them on the market have side effects, including a racing heart, feverishness, and headaches. But those biochemists know their stuff: down where it counts, you'll blow up like a balloon.

In fact, because these pills work so well, no matter which brand you're using, take only half a pill. Twice as much of the stuff is not twice as good, and you could end up with priapism, a painful condition involving unending erections that can be cured only through surgery. In fact, don't overdo any aspect of the penis-propping pills. Don't take them too often or try to make love beyond your tender parts' tolerance.

316 Should I wait for my girlfriend to have an orgasm every time?

Mysteriously but patently true, women don't have to have an orgasm to consider a sex act complete. Sometimes she is too tired, too distracted, or simply not in the mood. And frankly, you probably could not provide her one every time. A more important step is to make an effort each time to find out what her orgasm agenda is, either by asking or by gauging her response (or lack thereof) to your initial efforts to induce one, like rubbing her clitoris.

Trouble

You can't anticipate everything that goes wrong, but you'll be ahead of the game if you've anticipated the fact that something almost inevitably will. The coolest guy isn't the one who stays out of trouble, but gets out of it well. Here are a few suggested scenarios for when you need to come up with Plan B.

ON THE ROAD

317 **How do I fix a flat?**

Check your car's manual for the location of the spare tire, jack, and tire iron. If the manual is missing, look in the trunk (check under the carpet or behind a side panel). On some vehicles, the spare is often suspended under the rear of the car and has to be lowered using the jack handle to turn a bolt on the floor of the car. Once the tire is lowered, unhook it from its cable.

Make sure the car is on level ground so it doesn't rock when you jack it up. Pry off the hubcap with the thin end of the tire iron and loosen the lug nuts—the caps on the bolts securing the tire—with the other end. (You may need to give the tire iron a whack to get them started.) When the lug nuts are just loose, place the jack's lift carriage

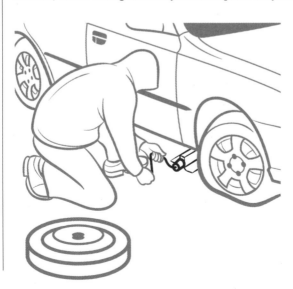

under the car just behind the front door on the side of the car where the flat is. The tire iron is the jack handle; pump or turn it until the flat tire is bearing no weight. (If you have no jack but can get a wrench to twist off the lug nuts, pull the tire opposite the flat one up onto the curb, or all the tires but the flat one onto the curb. This should free the tire up enough to take the tire off.)

Now finish loosening the lug nuts and put them somewhere close and safe. Pull off the tire and replace it with the spare. Put the lug nuts back on their bolts and tighten them by hand only, moving east to west, north to south, so the tire is balanced. Lower the jack all the way, and tighten the lug nuts snugly, again moving from bolt to bolt before giving them all a final twist.

Put away your tools, throw the flat tire into the trunk, and take it to a garage as soon as possible. Your spare is not meant to endure long-term use or very high speeds, so get it replaced immediately.

318 **What do the puddles under my car mean?**

If you see liquid in a parking spot you've just left, don't freak out; it could be the previous occupants' problem. Pull into another spot and see if the puddle forms there. If you have a large piece of paper, place it approximately where the original puddle was in relation to your car so you have something to show to your mechanic. Meantime, you can come up with a speedy diagnosis by noting the color of the liquid.

▶ Clear water near the front of the car probably means a leaky or split hose or a faulty water pump.

▶ Greenish puddles usually indicate a leak in the cooling system (you can verify that the drip is antifreeze by its sweet odor).

▶ Black, glossy goo is oil.

In all cases, when you've determined the liquid is coming from your car, you should get to a mechanic as soon as possible.

319 **What can I do when my car battery dies?**

You turn the key and the engine emits a series of quick ticks and your heart plummets into your stomach. Take a breath. It's possible that the cable connections to your battery are corroded: pop the hood and remove the connections to the battery posts. If you see yellow powder stuck to the posts and the clamps, you may have a bad connection. Rub away the yellow powder, avoiding getting it on your hands (it won't kill you, but if you do get it on your skin, make sure to wash it off), and reconnect the battery cables. If you still get the ticking noise, the battery needs a charge.

If you drive a standard, you can bypass the electric starter by "popping" the clutch. Open the driver's door and push on the door frame until you rock the car into forward motion. Recruit help or use the downslope of a hill if you need to. When the car is rolling nicely, hop into the driver's seat, shut the door, depress the clutch, and put the car in a low gear. Let the clutch out abruptly. The engine should catch and fire up. If not, repeat. Once the car is running, drive to a garage to find out why it wouldn't start.

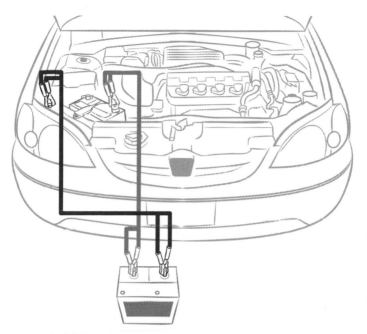

320 **How do I jump a battery?**

Got an automatic? You need to find another car and a pair of jumper cables. Park the live car's nose within a foot or so of the dead one with both cars in park, turn it off, and open both hoods. Find the red cable on the dead battery's red post, often marked with a plus sign. (Or jumper "plugs," which some new cars have instead, an equivalent to a surge protector for the car's onboard computer. Check your manual.) Clamp the other end of the red cable to the red post of the live car's battery. Now find the live car's black post, usually marked with a minus sign, and clamp the black jumper clamp to it. The other end gets clamped to the dead car's engine or engine frame, which looks completely inert and useless: i.e., not plastic, movable but a bolt or strut. Keep the cables themselves out of the engine.

Start the live car. Try to start the dead car. If it won't start, check that you've got the right connections and wiggle them to make sure the connection is firm. If the dead car still won't start, you need a tow.

321 What if a cop stops me for drunk driving?

The officer has already stopped you on probable cause for DWI. He or she does not have to get a positive reading on an alcohol-content-measuring test to take you in—so take the breath test. Refusing a breath test is grounds for suspending your license in most places; in some states you can go to jail. If you haven't been drinking, explain your erratic driving as best you can, but still take the Breathalyzer—and any other test the cop asks you to take.

322 Should I try to talk my way out of a ticket?

When an officer turns on the siren, his or her mind is probably made up. The only thing you can control is how many tickets you get. Be respectful, keep your language clean, and the cop may spare you citations for infractions like that burned-out brake light. If there are extenuating circumstances, explain them, but don't exaggerate and don't invent a dying mother whose bedside you're rushing to. He can check on these sorts of things.

If you were not in the wrong and can prove it, go before the judge to explain. It's even a good idea to go to court if you are guilty but can come up with some credible mitigating circumstances. A judge will often reduce a fine or points for your taking the effort to show up. Don't

323 HOW SHOULD I REACT WHEN I'M HEADING FOR AN ACCIDENT?

CHRIS COOK
former NASCAR driver, Chris Cook
Performance driving instructor

"Keep driving. The biggest mistake drivers make is to freeze up and let the accident happen. Instead, maximize your choices. Look where you want the car to go, not at the object you're heading for—if you're looking at the tree, you're going to hit it. Quickly identify the path of least resistance—a clear avenue away from the potential collision, or a ditch instead of a head-on collision. You won't always have a good choice, but you can pick the better outcome."

be Perry Mason or waste anyone's time, just explain the facts calmly and reasonably. Measure justice, however, against economics: it makes no sense to give up two hours' pay to save fifteen dollars on a fine.

324 What should I do when I see a speed trap?

By the time you see him, an officer already has your number on the speed gun. Resist the urge to hit the brakes hard. Officers prefer to see you slowing gradually to the legal limit. It shows respect, not panic, and will stand you in good stead.

1
2
3
4
5
6

325 **How do I handle a skid?**

When trying to regain control of a car, you want your front wheels aligned with the direction you are moving in. If the back end of your car begins to skid to the right, turn the steering wheel to the right. (This is what it means to "turn into a skid.") If you are headed for a collision, step on the brakes to slow the car, but if you're able, let the car slow on its own. In a manual transmission car, immediately push in the clutch to release the tires from 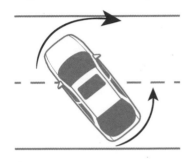 the engine; in an automatic, keep your foot off the pedals. When your back end stops sliding, steer gently back in the other direction.

326 **What's the best way to hit another car?**

If a car pulls out in front of you so that you have no choice but to hit it, aim for one of the wheels, preferably the one below the engine, the stiffest part of their car's frame, so that their car will tend to turn, not crush or split apart.

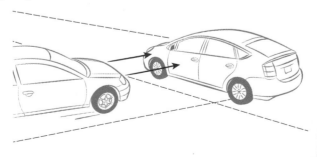

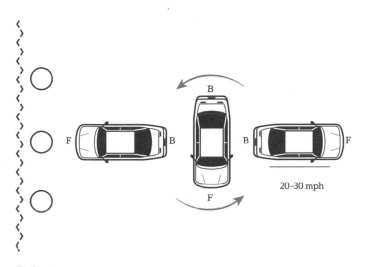

327 How do I evade a roadblock?

The most effective maneuver is a forward 180-degree spin. While moving 25 to 30 mph toward the roadblock, slip the car into neutral, and very decisively put the emergency brake on fully. As you do this, turn the wheel firmly to the right or left, at least a one-quarter turn. The car will spin in the direction in which the wheel is turned. When the car has completed the one-eighty, slip back into drive, release the emergency brake, and step on the gas. These nearly simultaneous steps take practice to execute; don't try it near other cars, people, or buildings.

If you have to ram the blocking car or structure to make your get-away, press the button on your dashboard to turn off your air bags. Slow down to about 10 mph to convince your assailant that you are stopping before accelerating again to 30 mph. Hit the barricade car on a wheel on the engine side, the stiffest part of its frame, to turn the car. Hitting a soft panel will only cause your vehicles to wrap together. Continue to accelerate until you have pushed it out of the way.

1
2
3
4
5
6

FISTICUFFS AND HANDCUFFS

328 **What can I do to avoid a fistfight?**

If you can outrun your opponent, law enforcement personnel recommend you try to do so. The bigger your opponent, the more likely it is that they won't be fast. Even a smaller opponent, however, is better avoided. A grown man need not fear teasing for shirking a brawl. The unintended consequences of violence are going to be worse than those of running.

When escape isn't an option, try to calm an imminently violent person by announcing repeatedly and rationally, "I don't want to fight you." This casts the other guy as the aggressor and may cause him to calm down. If a fight ensues anyway, bystanders are more likely to aid you, or tell your side of the story to the police.

329 **How do I punch someone?**

A badly thrown punch can hurt you as much as the other guy. Hold your fist so that the back of your hand is level with your forearm [a]; any bend in your wrist may cause your wrist to twist on impact, and reduce the force of your blow. Instead, punch directly from the

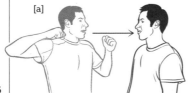
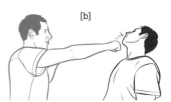

shoulder straight at the face [b]; don't swing your fist, drive it, aiming at a point a foot or so past his chin or mouth so you follow through after impact. The point is not to do maximum damage to your opponent's face but to knock him down. If you succeed, don't let him up; if he rises, push him to the ground and get a foot on his upper back, or punch him again.

330 **How do I win a street fight?**

Hit first. Street fights are usually preceded by threats, mutual insults, or a short pursuit; take these preliminaries as a chance to identify a leader of the group you're facing. As soon as you've made up your mind that flight is not an option, approach the leader and punch him forcefully in the mouth or nose with no further warning. Do not pull your arm back to wind up, which gives your target time to dodge. Do not take time to grab his clothing. In many cases the fall of the leader will induce his minions to walk away or make peace.

331 **How can I bring a troublemaker to the ground?**

Don't go out of your way to confront a guy who is verbally threatening you or others, but if his belligerence is verging on violence, you may want to attempt to neutralize him. He'll be expecting your intervention, but he's not expecting you to pull him toward you. Step close in and clap your left hand on his right shoulder [a]. At the same time, grab his left hand with your right and pull him forward strongly. In one motion throw his right hand behind his back [b] and take him flat to the ground.

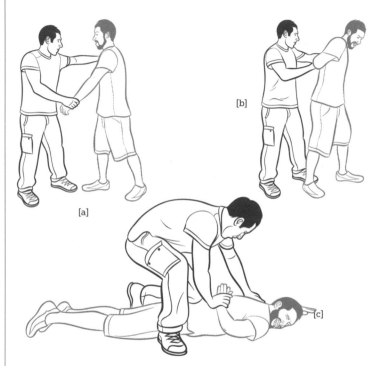

[a]

[b]

[c]

Keep upward pressure on his arm to inflict pain as he struggles, and let off the pain as he calms down [c]. Place a knee in the lower part of his back as a counterweight and you can use your free hand to phone for help.

332 **What can I do to avoid getting arrested?**

If you have advance notice that the police are on their way, calm yourself down, tuck in your shirt, comb your hair. Don't panic and don't

Ten classic rap albums every guy should know

- **RAISING HELL**
  Run-DMC (1986)

- **IT TAKES A NATION OF MILLIONS TO HOLD US BACK**
  Public Enemy (1988)

- **STRAIGHT OUTTA COMPTON**
  NWA (1988)

- **3 FEET HIGH AND RISING**
  De La Soul (1989)

- **THE CHRONIC**
  Dr. Dre (1992)

- **ENTER THE WU-TANG (36 CHAMBERS)**
  Wu-Tang Clan (1993)

- **READY TO DIE**
  The Notorious B.I.G. (1994)

- **ILLMATIC**
  Nas (1994)

- **ALL EYEZ ON ME**
  2Pac (1996)

- **THE MARSHALL MATHERS LP**
  Eminem (2000)

run. When the officer arrives, he or she will initially ask questions to determine whether a crime has been committed, and whether you are the one who committed it. As long as the officer is in this mode, be open and direct. Never get hotheaded or incommunicative. Listen carefully to the policeman's questions and answer them with a clear yes or no, which is very often plenty. As the officer gets a feel for what's going on, let him hear your side of the story. Needless to say, stay calm and treat the officer like a professional. Don't, however, be tempted to use profanity, which can itself be an arrestable offense.

333 **What should I do if I've been arrested?**

First, make sure you're under arrest. An officer may detain you without arresting you. Once the officer has put you under arrest, the game changes. His or her decision has been made, and nothing you say will overturn it. Ask the officer when you may call for legal help. Ask again when you are being processed at the police station or detention facility. Other than that, keep quiet and politely follow directions. Usually you'll be allowed as many phone calls as it takes to reach a lawyer or someone who can find you one. But in most locales, the number of phone calls you get, and the speed with which you get processed, can depend on how helpful you are.

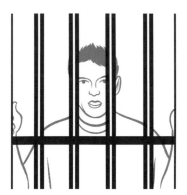

334 **How do I survive a night in jail?**

Unless you've committed an egregious offense, you will spend your evening in a relatively safe place: detention, not in a general-population jail. Despite what you see in the movies or hear in jokes,

Five modern comedy classics you should rent

CADDYSHACK (1980) The boobish Rodney Dangerfield hands over the reins of alternative comedy to the ironic, cool Bill Murray.

TOOTSIE (1982) Dustin Hoffman plays an actor who cross-dresses to get a role on a soap opera and falls in love with costar Jessica Lange.

WAYNE'S WORLD (1992) Mike Meyers and Dana Carvey glorify low-life midwestern dude-hood. The flick also explains the resurgence of both Queen's "Bohemian Rhapsody" and Rob Lowe's career.

THE BIG LEBOWSKI (1998) Jeff Bridges is the Dude, a guy who doesn't get why someone's trying to kill him.

OFFICE SPACE (1999) It may be that our current small-screen cubicle-comedy hits are inspired by this sleeper hit starring Jennifer Aniston. But its importance is secondary to its stupid laughs.

no harm is likely to come to you, from law enforcement or your fellow prisoners, in an overnight holding cell. That's not to say you'll be comfortable. Your patience and sense of fairness may well be sorely tested, and you shouldn't attempt to get any sleep even if you could. Nonetheless, adopt an attitude of quiet concentration, or, in the words of one police officer, "Don't run off at the mouth." Find a corner to yourself and don't look at your cellmates. If spoken to, be polite but cut off conversations and don't enter into any bargains or deals that other prisoners are interested in.

LOST AND FOUND

335 **How do I evade a manhunt?**

You have two main problems when being sought: humans recognize your appearance, including your clothes, facial markings, and car; dogs recognize your scent. Change your clothes, most immediately taking off anything you can be identified by and buying a whole new set if you can swing it without going to a store where you'd be exposed to cameras and possibly rack up a traceable transaction. Throw your cell phone away and ditch your car in favor of mass transit. Shave any facial hair or grow some. Wear hats until you can change your hairstyle. Stay away from places where humans congregate, heading for lonely rural areas far away from your usual haunts. Score cash early in your journey and don't use your plastic. Move after dark.

When being tracked by dogs, head for water and keep moving. Head downstream (so your scent is not trailing on the water's surface behind you) as far as you can stand.

336 **What do I do to stop a charging dog?**

A barking neighborhood bully will usually stop advancing on you if you step off its territory. If he pursues you on neutral turf, turn sideways while keeping your head turned to face the dog and yell, "No!" [a] Most yard dogs will respond to this common command. If this isn't one of them, change your stance to a low crouch [b] and, as the dog leaps at you, grab its neck behind the ears and pin it to the ground. Call for help.

You can tell immediately if the dog is trained in attack. He'll be

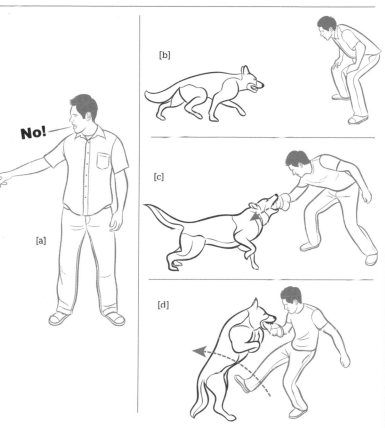

silent and approach very quickly. Take what time you have to wrap a jacket, sweater, or even a hat around your forearm [c]. Counter the dog's lunge with your own full weight as it arrives or you'll go over. As you defend, lodge your hand as far back in the dog's mouth as possible and grab the roots of its tongue [d]. Kick the dog smartly in the midsection and between its legs. If you have the nerve, place the thumb of your free hand at a corner of its eye and push. When the dog releases, keep it in front of you. Repeat if necessary.

1
2
3
4
5
6

337 **What do I do if I'm being followed?**

Behave slightly erratically—stop to look at a store window, a house, or a garden—and see if your tail tries to stick with you. If the person you suspect of following you stops (a store window makes for a convenient mirror to keep an eye on the person), walk on and stop again; if he or she stops again, it's likely you're being followed. If you want to make sure, walk around the block, and midway along the sidewalk, turn around abruptly but calmly and head in the other direction. If the tail turns with you, note the person's age, hair color, and height (measure visually against a building doorway or a street sign) so you can identify them to the police if need be.

The same method applies in a car. Turn on your right blinker, slow at the corner, and then continue straight. If you still have doubts, take two right turns and pull a U-turn midblock. On the highway, gradually slow down until you're doing 40 mph; anyone who's not following you will pass you within sixty seconds.

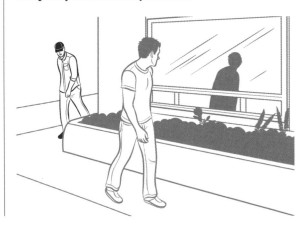

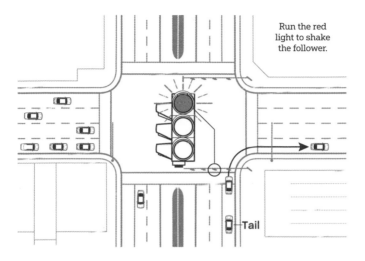

Run the red light to shake the follower.

Tail

338 How do I shake someone who is following me?

If your tail is a private investigator, the attempt to determine if he's tailing you will likely be enough; PIs would rather lose you and try again later than be discovered. If it's law enforcement—in which case, good luck, as they have the resources to have multiple agents as well as airborne surveillance. If you feel the person following you is a threat, whatever you do, don't go home; you don't want them to know where you live. Drive or walk to the nearest police station or squad car and explain your suspicions.

If you prefer to shake the tail yourself, put on your emergency blinkers and stop at the next red light. When the light turns green, stay put, and ignore the horns and yelling from other drivers. As the light turns red again, take off; the crossing traffic will prevent your pursuer from coming after you—not without exposing their agenda.

If, as you stall at the green, they drive around you and wait for you on the far side of the intersection, turn right.

In an extreme situation, stop your car in a crowded area, like a mall. Go into a busy department store—not a boutique—and find a fire alarm and pull it. In the resulting confusion, grab a jacket or other garment of a different color from the one you're wearing, and try to fit in with the crowd of shoppers leaving the store.

339 How do I communicate online securely?

If you're worried someone is tracking your electronic conversations, create an e-mail account on Gmail, Yahoo, or some other free service at an Internet café or at a public library. Put the information into an e-mail and save it as a draft without sending it. Then share the user name and password for that account with the person you want to communicate with (needless to say, share it via phone or snail mail). They can go onto the account and read it in the drafts folder.

340 What do I do if I'm lost in the wild?

Stop and just relax for a second. This isn't a Jon Krakauer book yet. You'll get out, but you need to stay calm. The tendency of a lost hiker is to try to hike his way out, expending energy he may want later and leading himself farther from the place friends or rangers will begin looking for him. Maintain your position and yell or fire a gun. (Two shots in close succession signal that you need help.) If you can start a fire, do it, and add green boughs to create smoke.

If you can climb a tree or a nearby hill to orient yourself or in the hope of seeing a camp or town, do so. Orient yourself to the sun's position or other landmark before you climb down. Start walking toward the civilized area while yelling for someone to notice you. Above all, stay calm. Panic wastes energy and breeds mistakes.

341 **How do I find a ski lost in a wipeout?**

Coming down the mountain was awesome . . . until you wiped out. But you dust yourself off, you're doing fine. No ski accident here. Uh, one problem? Where's your other ski?

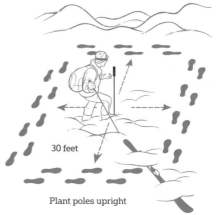

Plant your remaining ski—or a pole if you lost both skis—upright at the spot where you crashed. This will be the center of your grid. Walk in a straight line thirty feet in any direction—your ski is as likely uphill from you as down. Turn, walk

30 feet

Plant poles upright

another thirty feet and left again, until you arrive back at your marker. Now search the entire area you have enclosed with your steps, punching with your poles at the snow to widen the area of your coverage. If you don't find your ski, walk off another thirty-foot square box and search that one. At the farthest corner of each square, scan the snow far and wide.

1
2
3
4
5
6

Meanwhile, ask passersby if they have seen a ski, and to keep a lookout for a ski on their way down, in case yours took off for the lodge without you.

If you can't find your ski, it might be a good idea to invest in powder straps when you buy your new skis. The straps fly loose when your boot leaves the ski abruptly and trail atop the snow even if your ski burrows beneath.

342 **How do I right a canoe?**

You've capsized in your canoe. Maybe you were grandstanding for a friend, or maybe you just lost your balance, but the point is, you're in the water, and your boat is turned over. What do you do?

First, grab the paddles, or you'll be stranded even when you get the canoe right side up. Next take a moment to breathe. Consider whether you can swim ashore pulling the canoe behind you, as righting the canoe is arduous work. Getting back in is a challenge in itself. If you're too far away from shore, you can try one or more methods, depending on how heavy the canoe is and how many are in your group. (This entire process is much easier if you have life jackets on.)

If you're alone, heave yourself over the hull of the turtled canoe and grab the far gunwale (the top of the side of the boat). Rock backward, pulling the canoe with you.

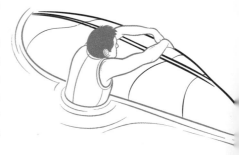

If you have a mate, duck under the canoe into the air pocket. Each of you takes one gunwale and on the count of three with a hard kick pushes up on one side of the canoe, flipping it upright.

If there is more than one canoe with you, bring the other's center perpendicular to the capsized one. All hands should lift the nose up and over the gunwale of the floating canoe and slowly pull the rest of the capsized canoe across it until the water has completely drained. Then flip the ailing canoe upright.

Take a break, hanging on the uprighted canoe, before trying to get back in. When you've caught your breath, come to the center of the canoe and, with one hand on the near gunwale, launch yourself over the boat with a big scissor kick to grab the far gunwale. Twist at the waist to sit down and pull your legs in. If you're with a friend, it's much easier. Have him or her hold on to the far gunwale as you scramble over yours.

343 **How do I prevent seasickness?**

That queasy feeling is your inner ear's inability to get a fix on the horizon, which seems to be tilting crazily. You can give your cochlea a fighting chance by staying on deck, where the far horizon is steady. (The fresh air, too, will help calm your stomach.) If you absolutely need to go on a boat, for a professional obligation, for example, a doctor can give you a patch you wear inconspicuously that pumps a small dose of motion-sickness drug into you.

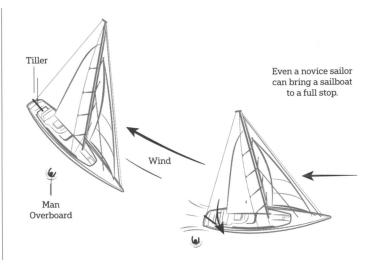

Tiller

Even a novice sailor can bring a sailboat to a full stop.

Wind

Man
Overboard

344 **How do I stop a sailboat?**

If you've never sailed, you're on a boat, and say your host falls overboard, here's what to do: Grab the tiller or wheel and steer the nose, or bow, of the boat directly into the wind. (If you're using a tiller—a large arm connected directly to the rudder—you push it in the *opposite* direction you want the bow to go.) As the bow comes into the wind, the sails will begin to flap and the boat to slow. Turn the wheel back to center to keep the boat facing the wind and the sails stalled. If you act quickly enough, your man overboard will be able to swim to catch up.

345 **What do I do for a blister during a hike?**

As soon as you feel a hot spot, stop and take care of it. At the camping store or many drugstores, you can score a foamy padding that you cut to surround the blister. But if you don't mind a little goo, and you're not near civilization, duct tape works just as well. Resist the urge to break a blister, leaving it open for infection to set in.

346 **How do I take care of a sunburn?**

The miracle of immediate relief is available in the form of Noxzema—the Original Deep Cleansing Cream—which takes the sting out mostly via its touch of menthol. But since Noxzema dries out the skin, it does more damage in the long run, and will induce you to peel like a snake. Better to treat the symptoms separately, and beneficially. For the painful touch, apply a lotion or spray containing lidocaine, a topical anesthetic, and pop a couple of ibuprofen to quell the inflammation. Then gently rub on some moisturizer that contains aloe and vitamin E.

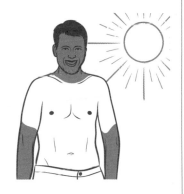

Another option: Brew a pot of tea and put a washcloth in with it. Wring out the washcloth, and apply to the surface of the burn. The tannins in the tea help soothe pain.

Acknowledgments

Thanks to Ingrid Abramovitch, who has a knack for making me step up my game, to Ann Bramson, Trent Duffy, Judy Pray, and everyone else at Artisan. To Tom Hardej for his steadfast work, my thanks as well. There is hardly a person I know who did not offer advice, help make a contact, or otherwise improve this book, but I'd like to acknowledge in particular Sarah Johnson for opening her generous and informative network to me. Of all the people who told me what to say, do, or think, I owe the greatest debt to Alice and to my family and my friends, who listened.

Index